PENGUI

THE FAT-STRIPPING DIET

Shane Bilsborough has a Master's degree in Science from Deakin University. He is the sports nutritionist for the MVP Football Academy at the South Melbourne Soccer Club and co-founder of the very successful lifestyle management company B Personal. In his capacity as a personal trainer, Shane has worked with elite athletes and corporate clients, helping them to achieve permanent weight loss. Shane has also worked as a top-billing international model. He now lives in Melbourne.

Shane can be contacted at www.bpersonal.com.au.

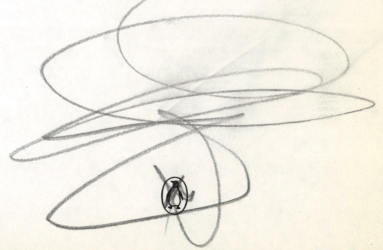

Shane Bilsborough

the fat stripping diet

PENGUIN BOOKS

Data for table on page 62 reprinted with permission by the American Journal of Clinical Nutrition © *Am. J. Clin. Nutr. American Society for Clinical Nutrition*

Penguin Books Australia Ltd
487 Maroondah Highway, PO Box 257
Ringwood, Victoria 3134, Australia
Penguin Books Ltd
Harmondsworth, Middlesex, England
Penguin Putnam Inc.
375 Hudson Street, New York, New York 10014, USA
Penguin Books Canada Limited
10 Alcorn Avenue, Toronto, Ontario, Canada M4V 3B2
Penguin Books (NZ) Ltd
Cnr Rosedale and Airborne Roads, Albany, Auckland, New Zealand
Penguin Books (South Africa) (Pty) Ltd
24 Sturdee Avenue, Rosebank, Johannesburg 2196, South Africa
Penguin Books India (P) Ltd
11, Community Centre, Panchsheel Park, New Delhi 110 017, India

First published by Penguin Books Australia Ltd 2001

1 3 5 7 9 10 8 6 4 2

Design and digital imaging by Susannah Low, Penguin Design Studio
Cover and author photograph by Bill Thomas
Typeset in 11/16 pt Minion by Post Pre-Press Group, Brisbane, Queensland
Printed and bound in Australia by McPherson's Printing Group, Maryborough, Victoria

National Library of Australia
Cataloguing-in-Publication data:

Bilsborough, Shane.
The fat-stripping diet.

Includes index.
ISBN 0 14 029531 3.

Low-fat diet. 2. Reducing diets. 3. Low-calorie diet.
4. Weight loss. I. Title.

613.25

www.penguin.com.au

A BIG THANK YOU for all the support given to me by: Elly Lanza of 'Virtue'; Tarik Kendja, Mark Stracey, Yevettski, Ralph Barba from 'The Four Diegos'; Michael Pitchner – one of the best fitness advisors around; 'Dr Delts' – Australian power-lifting champ Ian Webb; Berwick and Beverley Lourensz; Graeme Johnstone of Contemplative Design; Stephanie – the cover girl; Terrence and Francis Langendoen; Carl Clark; the Samoan giant – Fereti; Cherrie Miriklis of Flowers Vasette; Freda Miriklis and Andrew Christy of Sharetalk; Paul and Chrissie Velessaris; Patricia Johnson; Maggie, Kate and Danáe at Viviens; Dr Susan Holt; Mum and Neil, Dad and Lyn; Daniel Bilsborough; 'The Great One' Colin Delutis; and all the team at Penguin.

Thank you also to my brother Johann for all his efforts and help in the area of Human Movement and his sheer brilliance in this field, to Dr David Cameron-Smith from Deakin University who has been a great mentor to me, and to my awesome fiancée, Fiona, who has been there when this book was a mere thought and shared my joy, even through the hard times.

CONTENTS

Preface   ix

CHAPTER 1
Fats – the good, the bad and the ugly   1

CHAPTER 2
Carbohydrates, fibre and protein   23

CHAPTER 3
Sugar – is it fattening?   40

CHAPTER 4
How the body uses fat   49

CHAPTER 5
The energy cost of food   64

CHAPTER 6
Fat-stripping exercises   86

CHAPTER 7
The Fat-Stripping Diet   107

CHAPTER 8
Fat free – a leaner body   125

CHAPTER 9
Staying motivated   140

Appendices   147
References   166
Index   173

PREFACE

For many years I tried to understand the principles behind losing body fat. I failed, and came to the conclusion that the methods and theories I had read about were fundamentally flawed. I struggled to find a book that was written in simple terms that could help me understand the mechanisms behind losing fat and maintaining low but safe levels of fat. I was not the only person trying to find out how to lose body fat, as this was the burning question of the nineties and still is in the new millennium. Fad diet books that told me I could eat 'all the fat I liked' must have been someone's idea of a bad joke. I developed a 'beer gut', like many other people who eat large amounts of fat. I tried other books that told me not to eat carbohydrates because they raised insulin levels. Eat plenty of protein, they said! I couldn't concentrate at work, I had the jitters, my breath was bad, and I was dehydrated for much of the time. I later found out that protein raises insulin levels too, as much as and in some cases even more than carbohydrates. Diet books conveniently forgot to mention this. I realised that fat loss is a science that needs to be studied. I took the long way home to find out the answers. I went back to university, and three years later graduated with a Master's degree in Human Nutrition. My major studies were in food: how the body treats food; fat; fat metabolism; and fat metabolism during exercise.

The link between fat and how fat is metabolised in the body is basic information that is sadly lacking in many diet and exercise books. The factors that can actually help metabolise, or burn, fat are also poorly understood and hence many people are conned into believing fad theories. I questioned why so many diet books that omitted vital information on fat and fat metabolism were on the market.

A new approach

It became clear, as I ploughed through the diet books on the shelves in stores, that either the authors had no clear understanding of fat metabolism (as they were not qualified), or they simply chose to omit the facts that are pertinent to fat loss and concentrated on a short-term fad fat-loss theory. As I will show you, you don't have to be a doctor to understand these processes. In *The Fat-Stripping Diet*, the complex processes of fat metabolism or fat stripping are clearly defined and simply explained. This book contains what is taught at the best universities, by professional doctors of exercise and fat metabolism. I am not putting forward a fad theory. This is the real way fat is burnt.

Fat is responsible for fat storage. How would it make you feel to know that it would take a man of average height and weight 90–100 minutes of walking to burn off a fast food hamburger, and in this time he would need to walk about 8.5 kilometres? What if this same hamburger would take a woman 110 minutes to walk off? Would you think twice about eating it next time? In my experience as a personal trainer, I have seen how my clients react to hearing these statistics. I know I have certainly changed my attitude to eating foods high in fat, and so have many others, including my clients.

This book gives you a totally different perspective on fat. Are you tired of hearing 'How much fat's in that?', 'Five grams of fat is too much!', 'I've just eaten some chocolate, but I don't know how fattening it is'? *The Fat-Stripping Diet* will give you a clear understanding of how good and how bad fat is for you by converting excess fat (or surplus fat) into a distance you need to walk or run to burn it off. You will understand the real consequences of excess fat. This understanding in itself is a very powerful tool. The term 'excess or surplus fat' will also be clearly defined. The concepts behind fat loss are so straightforward – it's a wonder no-one has written about it before.

The diet alone can help you with effective fat and weight loss. By combining the diet with its associated fat-loss exercise program, you will decrease your body fat levels even further, and keep your weight off. These methods for fat loss were not 'thought up', but are the basics of human nutrition, exercise metabolism and physiology.

There are no tricks, creams, tablets, special lotions or

exercise equipment that you will need. Foods do not have to be eaten in combinations, in special ratios, or according to your hair colour or blood type. All I ask is that you bring with you the motivation and belief that you're going to make this work.

The actual eating program will hopefully be one that you will enjoy. The food prescribed is tasty, filling and there is plenty of it. In fact, if you follow the pattern correctly, you should be able to fit your foods of indulgence into the diet quite regularly. Preparation is the key here and you will be amazed at the amount you can accomplish and the weight you will lose if you put the time in to plan. Planning is an essential part of the Fat-Stripping Diet.

For the success of your diet you don't have to exercise initially, but by doing so, the amount of fat that you burn off will be greater. By including the exercise program in your lifestyle, you will increase the diet's effectiveness. The program is not exhausting, or difficult. There is a discrepancy in many of the diet books around about exactly what exercise is the best for fat loss. People assume that they have to push themselves until they drop to lose body fat. This is not correct. There are specific exercises and exercise intensities that must be met in order for your body to mobilise fat out of the fat cell, and to deliver this fat to your exercising muscles. Certain factors can affect how much fat you burn, and they are all explained in this book to help you achieve optimal fat stripping.

A better body for now and the future

Although most of us want to decrease our body fat now, it is also important to look at the bigger picture. If you can put some effective changes into your life today that will minimise your incidence of fat-related problems, then your quality of life will be enhanced. Your chance of getting a heart attack, stroke, diabetes or cancer can be dramatically decreased with these changes. The implications of the Fat-Stripping Diet can cascade through your whole life, and not just stop with fat loss. We all know the numerous benefits of good health. This diet can be your first positive step in the right direction.

You will reach the goals that you set with this book because this diet will finally answer all the questions you have ever asked about fat and how to get rid of it. It is my aim to equip you with all the information that you will ever need to fight fat and succeed. I know these methods work because not only are they the simple application of exercise physiology, metabolism and nutrition, but I have seen the satisfied looks on the faces of my clients. Remember the key to fat loss is planning, variety and patience.

I wish you luck in your endeavours to achieve fat and weight loss. I hope this book remains on your bedside table for many years to come.

Shane Bilsborough, 2001

FATS –
THE GOOD, THE BAD
AND THE UGLY

Key messages for this chapter

YOU WILL DISCOVER:

- what fat is
- the difference between fat and cholesterol
- why fats can be 'good' or 'bad'
- what hidden fats are
- the risks of eating too much fat
- what cellulite is
- what the future holds if we continue to eat as we do
- how to choose low-fat foods

What is fat?

We define fats as substances that are obviously fatty or oily in nature. Foods such as butter, cream, chocolate and anything deep-fried or junky are commonly associated with fat. Despite fats and oils being different in texture and taste, chemically they are very similar; for example, they are both insoluble in water. Fats are generally solid at room temperature whereas oils are liquid. A more scientific word for fat is 'lipid'.

1g of fat yields 38kj of energy

Fat is a very important part of the human body. In fact, we could not function without a certain amount of fat as the body uses it as a source for energy during the day. Small amounts of fat are used while you are sitting, standing or doing light tasks such as working or cleaning, and even while sleeping. However, the amounts of fat used in these instances are not significant enough to promote fat loss. The human body can readily burn approximately 41 grams of fat for women each day and 60 grams for men. Once you eat more than the maximum amount of fat needed for these daily processes, you have an amount of fat that is called surplus fat. This must be either stored or burnt off during exercise. Most people have enough fat stored in their bodies to walk 800–2400 kilometres!

The different types of fats found in the body are:
- structural fats
- storage fats
- metabolic fats
- fat-soluble vitamins
- transport fats

Structural fats

Fats are found surrounding almost every living cell in the body, protecting and adding reinforcement to the cell membrane. This protective layer of fat also acts as a barrier between the external environment of the cell and the cell itself. These fats may also be implicated by the conversion of carbohydrate to structural fat when a person overeats. (This is not to be confused with storage fat.)

Storage fats

Storage fats supply the body with an abundant source of fuel. The specific storage site for fat is in a tissue called the adipose tissue, which can be found throughout the body. When you have too much fat in your diet, it gets stored. The more fat you eat, the greater this storage fat becomes, and the harder it is to work it off. These storage fats have two and a half times more energy (kilojoules) than carbohydrates and take up less space than carbohydrates. These fats also provide the body with insulation. This is the type of fat that any weight management program aims to lose. We don't need an excess of storage fat.

Metabolic fats

This is a term that refers to fat which, once digested, is converted to substances that are chemically important in our bodies, such as hormones and enzymes. These fats maintain the body's metabolism. The metabolism describes all the ongoing and essential activities of the body that we sometimes take for granted. These activities use energy and they include:

- keeping the heart beating and pumping blood around the body
- breathing
- breaking down food, transporting and storing it
- producing new cells and removing old ones
- producing enzymes and hormones
- filtering blood through the kidneys

Fat-soluble vitamins

One of the most important points about fat intake is that fat contains fat-soluble vitamins. These vitamins are A, D, E and K and are essential. They may be stored in the liver, or the fat tissue.

Transport fats

Fats must be transported from the intestine through the bloodstream to their storage sites. They are transported through the body, or 'piggybacked' through the bloodstream, on a specific type of transport fat called lipoprotein. Lipoprotein is actually a special form of cholesterol (see page 7). Fats are constantly moving through the body, from storage sites to the liver, where they can be broken down to form steroids and hormones, and to active or exercising muscles, where they can be burnt as fuel.

Different types of fats found in food

As we have seen, there are different types of fats found in the body and they all have different functions. The fat in food is also very varied and can be somewhat confusing for many people. We hear so much about 'good' fats and 'bad' fats, but what does it all mean? Does it mean that if a fat is considered good, we can eat as much of it as we want and not get fat? Does it mean that we can pour copious amounts of olive oil on our dressing and we will have better health because of it, or is there more to the story? Are there limits to the amount of good fats that we can eat? Does eating too much good fat make us fat? These questions are answered by looking at the following classes of fats:

- essential fatty acids
- cholesterol
- saturated, polyunsaturated and mono-unsaturated fats

Essential fatty acids

In 1929, two American nutritionists fed their laboratory rats a fat-free diet. What they found as a result of this was quite startling. The deficiencies that these rats developed could be prevented by the addition of certain fats, later termed essential fatty acids or EFAs. From this research it was established that these fats have many vital functions in the human body. A deficiency of EFAs can lead to the rupturing of cells, allowing small molecules and water into the cell. This loss of the cell function decreases the ability of the cell to produce and function at an optimal level. EFAs are also involved in:

- muscle contraction
- blood clotting
- control of blood pressure
- prevention of scaly dermatitis
- production of hormones
- function of the nervous tissue of the eye and brain

The body does not have the ability to make these fats and so they must be obtained through eating certain foods. There are two main types of EFAs: linoleic acid and linolenic acid. Linoleic acid is found in vegetable oils such as maize, sunflower, canola and safflower oil. Linolenic acid is found in green leafy vegetables such as spinach, cabbage and lettuce, in vegetable oils such as soybean, sunflower and olive oil, and fish. Possible external signs of EFA deficiency are the appearance of skin lesions and dermatitis. It is recommended that the daily intake of linoleic acid is 3–5 per cent of the total energy intake (9–14 grams) and that of linolenic is 0.5–1 per cent of the total energy intake (3 grams). In more specific terms, three-quarters of a tablespoon of sunflower oil and half a teaspoon of olive oil per day will meet the essential fatty acid requirements of the human body. If your intake of these fats is in excess of the recommended daily amount, then they will be stored as body fat.

Cholesterol

Cholesterol is produced naturally in the body, namely in the liver and in most cells, and is essential for good health. It is involved in the production of sex hormones and bile, which has an important role in the digestion of fat, aiding the absorption of fat into the bloodstream. Bile helps dissolve fat much in the way detergent dissolves fat from a greasy plate.

Humans produce approximately 1 gram (less than half a teaspoon) of cholesterol daily, which is all the cholesterol the body needs to function optimally. There is no need to add extra cholesterol to our diet, although many foods common to the Western diet, such as dairy products and red meat, contain high levels of cholesterol. Specific cholesterol particles called lipoproteins are found in human blood. The two main lipoprotein particles are low-density lipoprotein (LDL) and high-density lipoprotein (HDL). Both particles are produced naturally by the body and form a harmonious relationship. They are involved in the delivery of cholesterol and fat to the cells and liver. The LDLs, or 'bad' cholesterol, deliver cholesterol to sites around the body, such as artery walls, while the HDLs, the 'good' cholesterol, collect this deposited cholesterol and take it back to the liver, where it is broken down to produce bile. There are several ways in which we can disrupt this balance: smoking, eating foods that contain cholesterol and eating saturated fats all increase the number of LDL particles in the blood. When there is an excess of LDLs in the body, they lead to the accumulation of cholesterol-rich droplets on artery walls, making the arteries very narrow. This can increase the risk of heart disease. If a small piece of this cholesterol becomes dislodged from the artery wall, then it can circulate to the arteries of the heart and cause a blockage of blood flow, resulting in a heart attack. Similarly if these particles block the flow of blood to the brain, then a stroke eventuates.

The HDL is responsible for taking cholesterol back to the liver, thereby removing it from the blood. It is of benefit to your health to have a substantial level of HDL particles in your bloodstream and this is something you can control. The levels of LDLs and HDLs can increase or decrease according to the type and amount of food that you consume. Eating foods that are high in cholesterol, such as butter, cream, eggs, cheese, meat, brains, liver and offal, will increase your level of bad cholesterol (LDL), while eating small amounts of foods such as olive oil, sunflower oil and soybean oil will decrease it. Remember that plant foods such as fruits and vegetables contain no cholesterol. Eating plenty of fruit, oats, cereals, breads, rice and legumes will actually decrease your bad cholesterol, and regular exercise can increase your level of good cholesterol (HDL). If you are unsure about your cholesterol levels, a simple blood test will reveal all you need to know. Before embarking on any weight-loss or exercise program, it is a good idea for your doctor to check your cholesterol and blood pressure levels. This way you or your personal trainer can determine the best intensity for you to begin at, and you can then monitor your progress with regular medical check ups.

CHOLESTEROL LEVELS IN FOOD

FOOD	AMOUNT OF CHOLESTEROL (mg)
1 slice chopped liver, fried	234
1 medium egg	206
6 king prawns	190
160 grams crayfish	180
200 grams veal	158
2 sausages	76
2 rashers bacon	52
1 tablespoon butter	36
1 cup full-cream milk	35
1 cube cheese	16
fruits	0
vegetables	0

The different types of household fat

To illustrate examples of the three types of fats that are most common in our diets, we will use butter, margarine and olive oil. They represent (in order) saturated fat, polyunsaturated fat and mono-unsaturated fat.

Saturated fat

This term refers to the chemical composition of the fat. Saturated fats increase LDLs and decrease HDLs in the bloodstream, increasing the risk of heart disease. Some scientific evidence suggests that they also stay in the fat cells longer. This means that they go into the fat cell first but are removed from the fat cell last. Needless to say, foods rich in saturated fat should be avoided.

Butter, a saturated fat, has been shown to increase bad cholesterol levels (LDL). Other saturated fats are cream, cheese and full-cream milk. Saturated fats such as coconut oil and palm oil are used extensively in the food industry, so while you think you may be eating a healthy, low-fat stir-fry from a noodle bar, you could actually be consuming large amounts of 'hidden' fats. When you are dining out it is difficult to know exactly how your food is cooked, or how much oil has been used but whenever possible, ask! These hidden fats sabotage healthy eating and if you are trying to lose fat, this is one area where you can easily reduce your fat intake. When you are in the supermarket, read the label to find out if the product that you are about to purchase contains saturated fat, and if so how much. In these small ways you can take control of how much fat you eat and in what form you eat it.

Polyunsaturated fat

Polyunsaturated fats are considered to be 'good' fats in small amounts because they have the ability to lower bad

> ## EICOSANOIDS
> These hormone-like compounds are produced from omega-3 fatty acids, which are found in abundance in marine animals, including fish. They are primarily involved with regulating blood pressure and blood clotting. Specifically, these compounds lower blood cholesterol, and reduce the tendency for the blood to clot.
>
> Other compounds produced from omega-3 fatty acids are prostaglandins and thromboxanes. These compounds have a similar role to eicosanoids.

cholesterol levels (LDL). Sunflower oil, soybean oil and green leafy vegetables all contain polyunsaturated fats. Green leafy vegetables also contain small amounts of essential fatty acids (see pages 5–7). These EFAs are not stored as fat, but are used to provide energy for the body's metabolism. Shellfish also contains polyunsaturated fats. (Interestingly, shellfish contains quite high levels of cholesterol yet it is extremely low in fat.) Margarine is another example of polyunsaturated fat. However, during the manufacturing process some of the fats contained in margarine (and other polyunsaturated fat products) are converted to trans-fatty acids. These trans-fatty acids are thought to increase bad cholesterol levels (LDL), but are present in such low levels, if at all, in Australian products, so using small amounts of margarine can be beneficial. The amounts of trans-fatty acids in certain foods are detailed on the nutritional label, so check thoroughly before purchasing.

Mono-unsaturated fat

Like polyunsaturated fats, mono-unsaturated fats also have the ability to lower bad cholesterol (LDL) and are hence considered to be 'good' oils. A regular consumption of olive oil is beneficial in lowering LDLs and decreasing the risk of heart disease. Avocados, olives, eggs, fish and chicken also contain mono-unsaturated fats. Although it has been advocated that some of these oils and fats are beneficial to our health (as they are low in cholesterol), they are still fattening when consumed in excess.

If we were to round up the fats, both the good and the bad,

FISH OR FISH OIL SUPPLEMENTS?

The answer is definitely fish. Fish contains substances called long-chain fatty acids, also known as omega-3 fish oils, which can actually raise the HDL levels in the blood. Eaten a few times per week, fish should supply you with adequate amounts of omega-3 fatty acids. When cooked properly it is healthy and low in fat and contains many important vitamins and minerals. Regulating your diet to eat less saturated fat and moderate amounts of mono- and polyunsaturated fats, such as in olive oil and green leafy vegetables, may be just as beneficial as taking omega-3 fish oil supplements.

---

that we have so far described, we would find that one tablespoon of butter has almost the same amount of fat as one tablespoon of margarine, as would be the case with similar amounts of olive oil and sunflower oil. This is a key point to remember: while some of these fats affect cholesterol levels for better or for worse, none of these fats, even the good ones, actually makes you lose weight. By all means use healthy mono-unsaturated and polyunsaturated fats, such as extra-virgin olive oil and sunflower oil, in your cooking, but remember to use them sparingly as they do add extra fat and energy to your diet. As men and women respectively use 60 grams and 41 grams of fat each day (see page 2), of which 12–17 grams is essential fatty acids, then the rest of the fat should come in the form of 'good' fats.

> All oils, whether
> 'good' or 'bad',
> are still fattening
> when eaten in excess.

The following table shows the similarities of fat content in oils of very different origins. The table reveals no real difference at all amongst the oils. The only minimal difference is in canola oil, which has 0.2 grams of fat less per tablespoon. Generally, the nutritional panel on the label will show you the exact amount of fat contained in each bottle of oil. It is very useful to familiarise yourself with these figures and to read the label before you buy a certain product.

FAT CONTENT OF OILS

OIL	AMOUNT OF FAT IN 1 TABLESPOON (grams)
olive oil	14
extra-light olive oil	14
extra-virgin olive oil	14
grapeseed oil	14
peanut oil	14
sunflower oil	14
canola oil	13.8

Health risks of a high-fat intake

If you regularly eat foods that are high in fat then you are putting your health at risk. As we have previously discussed, a high-fat diet can lead to an excess of storage fat, making you overweight or even obese. Statistics show that over half the population of the USA is overweight. Data from 1997 showed that in America, a person died from heart disease every 33 seconds, totalling 2600 deaths from heart disease every day. Nearly 12 000 000 suffered from either a stroke or heart attack annually. The 1995 Australian National Health Survey found that roughly 45 per cent of all adults were either overweight or obese. In Australia, a person dies from heart-related problems every six minutes. This is an alarming figure. Statistics also show that in Australia more than one-third of the food we eat

> ## HOW MUCH FAT?
> The human body stores about 9000 grams of fat. This provides enough energy for a person to walk continuously for 11 days or to run continuously for 4 days.

is in the form of fat. In the United Kingdom, over 20 per cent of eighteen-year-olds are overweight, and future projections for an overweight populace are certainly cause for concern. What makes this even more bizarre is the fact that the low-fat-food industry is booming, as are sales of exercise machinery. Books on health and wellbeing top the number-one bestseller lists around the world, yet many people are still dangerously overweight and becoming ever more unfit and unhealthy.

Fat storage in men and women

Men tend to store fat on their abdominal region, whereas women predominantly store fat on their hips and thighs. Fat can also be stored on the stomach, back of the arms and back. Although there are many theories behind this, it all boils down to genetics and hormones. It is thought that in hunter–gatherer times when men would go out on long journeys in search of food, a little abdominal fat provided extra energy for these long journeys. These hunters survived better than their thinner, leaner cohorts, and hence this genetic trait has been passed down from generation to generation. Men produce testosterone, which promotes the storage of fat on the stomach or central trunk region. However, this fat can be removed quite easily.

Storage of fat in the stomach region and a diet high in fat increase the risk of:

- lower-back pain, joint pain
- shortness of breath
- high blood pressure
- excessive blood cholesterol (hyperlipidaemia)
- diabetes
- heart disease
- stroke
- colon cancer

The female body produces oestrogen, which promotes the storage of fat on the hips, thighs and buttocks. For women it was found that in times of famine, those who possessed a larger amount of fat on their hips and thighs survived. Hence this genetic blueprint has been passed down to the women of today. The storage of fat on the hips and thighs is essential and protective during pregnancy, as it ensures a long-term supply of energy. Unlike the fat on the stomach, this fat is hard to burn off.

Cellulite

The dimpling of the skin on the thighs and buttocks is commonly referred to as cellulite. Cellulite afflicts women more frequently than men. Although many therapies presume that cellulite is caused by abnormal fat or fat that contains toxins, the basic development of cellulite has not yet been clearly established. Cellulite is just fat that has moved out of its fat cell. Tissue can grow over these fatty areas, and when pulled tight it can give a lumpy appearance. It seems that moving fat from the lower part of the body is more difficult than moving it from the upper body. This may be due to the fact that women are genetically and/or hormonally predisposed to storing fat on their legs and buttocks. It seems, however, that the fat itself is no different from any other fat, so with a solid exercise program and a sensible eating pattern cellulite can be mobilised and used as fuel just as fat anywhere else can be. Interestingly, people who crash diet and lose weight too quickly still retain cellulite around their bodies.

There are no miracle cures or creams that will rid your body of cellulite. Firming lotions, hot spas, cellulite creams or deep-tissue massage do nothing to decrease the body's amount of cellulite. The secret to cellulite mobilisation is knowing how to correctly burn fat as a fuel during exercise.

THE FALSE PROMISES OF FAT BUSTERS

- deep-tissue massage that rubs out cellulite
- pineapples that help burn cellulite
- plastic wraps that make cellulite float to the surface of the skin
- special creams that can be rubbed into the skin to burn cellulite
- fat-burning tablets
- amino acid powders that burn fat and cellulite

Can certain foods burn fat?

Popular belief has it that if you eat certain foods, or specially prepared herbs, your body can burn more fat. Once again, this concept couldn't be further from the truth. Cons such as this rely on clever marketing tricks to mislead people into purchasing various products. In order for a product to truly stand by its claim, it needs to undergo careful scientific tests. These tests are necessary to determine whether the substance actually works under controlled conditions, to find out whether it is safe or toxic, and to understand what its optimal dosage is. Testing is also necessary to see whether the product has been contaminated by impurities in the manufacturing and storing process. If a product does not meet these criteria, then it is difficult to assess or believe its worth. You wouldn't buy a new car unless you could see that it worked, and it came with a warranty. Rigorous scientific testing is like your warranty.

Products claiming to have fat-burning properties may use similar ploys to those used by companies selling cellulite cures. To date there is very little evidence of 'natural' substances burning significant amounts of fat to aid in weight and fat loss. The December 1999 *Australian Medical Journal* reviewed all the available evidence for the effectiveness of popular fat, cellulite and weight-loss non-prescription supplements. Some of the products tested included:

- hydroxycitric acid, or HCA, found in the rind of an exotic citrus fruit
- hot peppers or chillies, containing capsaicin

- caffeine/guarana, from the leaf of the South American vine *Paullinia cupana*
- L-carnitine, an amino acid powder
- chitosan, an amino sugar taken from the powdered shells of prawns and crabs
- chromium picolinate
- *Fucus vesiculosus*, found in various products such as Cellasene
- ginkgo biloba, found in the leaves of the maidenhair tree
- pectin
- grapeseed extract
- horse chestnut
- St John's wort
- milk thistle
- fat-burning tablets
- pyruvate

The study concluded that there was no evidence that these substances were effective in reducing fat/cellulite or weight. If you are ever in doubt about the validity of a product with this type of claim, check with your local university or a certified nutritionist.

What about 'light' foods?

There has been a lot of confusion about the terms used to describe the fat content of foods. For example, the word 'light' or 'lite' has been used on various oils. This type of label gives the consumer the impression that the product is low in fat, but this may not always be the case. 'Light' has been used in some circumstances to mean light in colour and taste. Reading the nutritional panel on the label to check the fat content will clarify whether 'light' does actually mean low-fat. 'Low-fat', 'light', 'diet' and 'skim' products may well be lower in fat than their full-fat or full-flavoured counterparts, but comparing the nutritional values will reveal that the fat content of low-fat cheese, for example, is still quite high. Generally speaking, however, low-fat products are lower in fat than full-fat products. It is important to remember that although you may always consume low-fat products, the amount of fat in your daily diet can unknowingly add up. Just because it is low in fat doesn't mean you should have twice as much! An interesting exercise is to compare the differences between low-fat foods and their full-fat counterparts.

LOW-FAT VS HIGH-FAT

FOOD DESCRIPTION	FAT PER 100 g SERVING (grams)
natural yoghurt (Jalna)	4.3
natural yoghurt (Jalna), skim	0.1
yoghurt (Ski)	4.0
light yoghurt (Ski)	0.9
coconut cream	58.0
light coconut cream	17.0
coconut milk	17.0
light coconut milk	6.0
cheese, super slices (Bega)	27.0

LOW–FAT VS HIGH–FAT – *continued*

FOOD DESCRIPTION	FAT PER 100 g SERVING (grams)
So Light cheese (Bega)	15.0
Super Slim cheese (Bega)	10.0
light cheese (Kraft)	16.0
extra-light cheese (Kraft)	9.5
fat-free cheese (Kraft)	2.7

supermarket survey 20.09.99

FAT CONTENT OF MILKS

FOOD DESCRIPTION	FAT PER 250 g SERVING (grams)
full-cream milk	9.5
reduced-fat milk	2.3
high-calcium milk	0.38
skim milk	0.1
Skinny milk	0.25
Big M	7.8
REV	3.0
Light Start	2.5
Breaka	9.3
Breaka lite	2.3
soy premium	8.5
low-fat soy milk	2.3

supermarket survey 20.09.99

The differences in coconut milk, for example, are quite remarkable. Coconut cream has nearly three times more fat than its low-fat version, and three times more fat than coconut milk. Light coconut milk, on the other hand, has nearly ten times less fat than coconut cream. These differences can be established by simply going to the supermarket armed with a pen, paper and a pocket calculator. This kind of knowledge is just part of the planning process that will help you strip fat and keep it off.

SUMMARY:

- fats have an important role in the body
- we need to eat a certain amount of fat
- too much fat gets stored
- there is no difference between cellulite and fat
- fat and cholesterol are related
- different fats can affect your cholesterol levels and, in the long term, your health
- the human body can use up or metabolise roughly 41 grams of fat for women and 60 grams of fat for men each day
- nutritional labelling is important and can help you to make more informed choices about food

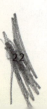

CARBOHYDRATES, FIBRE AND PROTEIN

Key messages for this chapter

YOU WILL DISCOVER:

- the importance of carbohydrates, fibre and proteins in the diet and the different roles they play
- how carbohydrates are broken down to glucose
- why the brain and nervous system functions primarily on carbohydrates
- how fibre can decrease the risk of colon cancer
- the problems with low-carbohydrate diets
- how the body can cannibalise protein to make glucose

What are carbohydrates?

Carbohydrates are chains of glucose units chemically joined together. Carbohydrates are found in almost all plant products but they are not present in significant amounts in animal products, except milk. The prime objective of carbohydrates is to supply energy to the body. Once eaten, carbohydrates are broken down into simple units of glucose. There are two basic types of carbohydrates: complex and simple. Complex carbohydrates are broken down slowly to release glucose into the blood over a long period of time. Examples of complex carbohydrates are cereals and grains, such as pasta, rice and mixed grains, and root vegetables such as potatoes, sweet potatoes and cassava. Simple carbohydrates are broken down relatively quickly and hence release larger amounts of glucose into the blood in a short period of time. Examples of simple carbohydrates are honey, malt, sugar and glucose itself. The functions of carbohydrates, both complex and simple, include:

- keeping the heart beating and pumping blood around the body
- breathing
- breaking down food, transporting and storing it
- producing new cells and removing old ones
- filtering blood through the kidneys while you are asleep
- producing hormones and enzymes

In the small intestine carbohydrates are broken down to glucose and smaller glucose chains. These glucose units are then transported to storage sites around the body, and stored in the liver and muscle cells. Stored glucose is known as glycogen. The amount of glucose that can be stored in the body is remarkable, yet these stores can be depleted very quickly because glucose is the primary energy source for the human body. In muscles, for example, the body can store 400–500 grams of glucose. This is the equivalent of twenty-two slices of bread or twenty-five small to medium-sized potatoes. In the liver cells the body can store a further 70 grams of glucose. This is the equivalent of four slices of bread or four medium-sized potatoes. Hence, in total, there is room for the equivalent of twenty-six slices of bread or twenty-nine small to medium potatoes in the body.

Carbohydrates are essential for our energy needs. Although it may appear that the body can store vast amounts of carbohydrates, it must be clearly understood that these stores can easily run very low and are rarely at full-storage capacity. If you miss breakfast, for example, then not only will you feel weak and lethargic, you could also feel irritable and cranky, and have a low concentration span. This is primarily because your body has been slowly using glucose during the night, and during your early-morning activities. Your blood glucose levels have run low, meaning that the amount of glucose stored in your liver and muscles is very low. Other symptoms of a low-carbohydrate intake are headaches, from low blood sugar levels, and constipation. Most of the time some carbohydrate, such as a sandwich, will quickly fix this. The more complex the carbohydrate you eat, the longer your energy will last. Considering that your brain needs glucose on a minute-to-minute basis, as does your nervous system, it is unwise to go for too long without eating a proper meal.

We can use breakfast as an example to show how simple and complex carbohydrates differ. If you have some fruit for breakfast, you will get a relatively quick burst of energy that will only last for a short period of time. You have consumed what is termed simple carbohydrates (also called simple sugars). If, on the other hand, you have eaten two to three pieces of toast, you will have longer lasting energy because the body breaks this bread down into glucose over a few hours. You may not feel hungry for a while after this type of breakfast. Satiety, the feeling of 'fullness', is a common sensation after eating carbohydrates. After eating fruit, however, you will feel hungry very shortly after breakfast, and you may also develop the symptoms of low blood sugar as previously described.

How much carbohydrate should I be eating?

Carbohydrates should supply up to 60 per cent of your energy. Qualified nutritional experts recommend a carbo-hydrate intake of roughly 300–400 grams per day for males and 300 grams per day for females. The remainder of our energy should come from 20–25 per cent proteins and 15–20 per cent fat. When you consider that during an hour of intense weight training a woman can use 115 grams of glucose and a man can use 150 grams, you realise that an adequate carbohydrate intake is essential.

Carbohydrates are good for you

In order to digest, break down, transport and store carbohydrates as glucose, the body uses roughly 10 per cent of the energy of the incoming food. Think of this in terms of the cost of storage. For example, in order for the body to store three small-sized potatoes (50 grams of carbohydrate), it will cost the body 10 per cent of 50 grams, which is 5 grams. Therefore, 45 grams of the carbohydrate in the potatoes is converted to glucose and stored as glycogen. The other 5 grams of carbohydrate is used by the body for energy to help pay for the storage of the 45 grams. Carbohydrates are better for you than fats because your body can burn more energy eating carbohydrates than it can by eating fat. This is called the thermic effect of food and it represents the huge advantage that carbohydrate has over fat. If, for example, you ate 50 grams of fat, it would cost only 3 per cent to store this fat as fat. Therefore, 1.5 grams of fat is used in storing 48.5 grams as fat. As you will see in Chapter 5, it requires no walking or running to burn off 45 grams of glucose. To walk off 48.5 grams of fat, however, is very time-consuming.

Brain food

Glucose is the fuel that allows the brain and nervous system to function. The brain has a high metabolic rate and needs

130–200 grams of glucose per day to function normally. There are relatively few blood capillaries around the brain, therefore oxygen, transported in the blood, is also highly prized by the brain, which is extremely sensitive to anoxia, a lack of oxygen. As glucose can be produced in the body without oxygen, this makes glucose an ideal energy source for the brain, as fat cannot be produced in the absence of oxygen. It seems that even during periods of starvation, one of the major aims of the body is to supply glucose to the brain. The brain cannot store glucose and it therefore depends on glucose from the intake of carbohydrates from your diet. In an extreme situation, if the level of glucose in the blood should fall below a certain level, even for a short space of time, then irreversible brain damage can occur.

Fibre

It is well documented that a diet high in fibre has a long list of benefits. It has also been strongly suggested by nutritionists and doctors that we should adhere to a diet that contains unrefined, high-fibre carbohydrates. In doing so we protect ourselves against many prevalent Western health problems, such as heart disease and colon cancer. In simple terms, fibre is the indigestible portion of food of plant origin, such as the skin of an apple. Our bodies cannot break down the bulk of these skins because we lack the specific enzymes needed to do so. Fibre, therefore, passes through the body relatively quickly, taking digested foods and water out of the body with it. Constipation can be a common indication of insufficient fibre in your diet. Foods such as legumes, baked beans, peas, broccoli, bananas and pears are all good sources of fibre. Cereals and grains are also high in fibre. They can be found in complex carbohydrates such as breads, particularly dark rye bread and wholemeal bread. High-fibre diets are followed in such areas as rural Africa, and their level of heart disease and colon cancer is low as a result.

Healthy weight control

High-fibre foods may also help to regulate a person's weight, as many high-fibre carbohydrate-rich foods don't contain fat. It makes sense, then, that replacing fatty foods with fibrous foods decreases the amount of ingested fat and cholesterol. Less fat means less fat storage and more energy expended by the body to break down high-fibre carbohydrate-rich foods. If high-fibre carbohydrates such as bread, cereals, rice and pasta are eaten instead of fatty, oily foods, then this can promote weight loss. Fibrous foods absorb more water than their non-fibrous counterparts and can therefore leave a person feeling full once eaten. Foods high in fibre also contain many essential vitamins and minerals, and contain fewer kilojoules per mouthful than high-fat foods.

Health benefits

In the developed world, cancer is the second largest cause of death among men and women. Colon cancer is in the top three of the list of fatal cancers. A diet high in fibre can significantly reduce the risk of colon cancer. High-fibre carbohydrates pass through the body quickly and thus the so-called 'transit time' of food is quite short. As previously mentioned, the fibre drags the digested food contents of the intestines with it, decreasing the time that the colon is exposed to any potential carcinogen in the food.

High-fibre diets are also strongly recommended to decrease the risk of heart disease, usually caused by high levels of cholesterol. It has been suggested that some fibres can bind to bile acids in the gut and drag cholesterol out of the gut with these bile acids. This can decrease the amount of bad cholesterol (LDL) in the blood. Oats, beans and lentils are good sources of this fibre.

As high-fibre complex carbohydrates slowly release glucose into the blood, insulin levels rise only to moderate levels. This is particularly useful if you are a diabetic and need to control your blood sugar levels.

How much fibre should I eat?

You should include roughly 30 grams of fibre per day in your diet. This figure is part of your total carbohydrate intake, which provides 60 per cent of the body's energy, for the day. If you were to eat two bananas (6 grams), one apple and one pear (7 grams), one bowl of cereal (7 grams) and one bowl of wholemeal pasta (10 grams) in a day, then you would meet all your fibre requirements. The amount of fibre that you should be eating every day is taken into consideration in the Fat-Stripping

Diet 7-Day eating plan (see pages 154–9), so you certainly don't need to stringently measure exact amounts.

Can I eat too much fibre?

You certainly can! People who eat excessive amounts of fruit and vegetables can experience stomach pains, flatulence and diarrhoea. In this case, you risk losing water-soluble vitamins as well as fluid. Too much fibre can also result in a loss of valuable minerals. Phytic acid, which is found in the husks of seeds, grains and legumes, can bind to minerals such as copper, magnesium, iron, zinc and calcium and remove them unnecessarily from the body. A loss of these minerals can lead to deficiencies that have a long list of problems of their own.

Protein

Sources of protein include red meat, chicken, fish, eggs, cheese, milk and some vegetables such as peas. Eating good-quality protein is important because protein is second only to water in its abundance in the body. Protein is responsible for, or involved in, the following functions:

- structure of cell membranes
- growth and repair of muscle tissue
- hair and nail growth (referred to as inert proteins)
- enzymes and hormones
- transporting proteins
- connective tissue such as elastin and collagen
- immune-system antibodies

Protein is broken down into amino acids, which are responsible for the production of enzymes, hormones and the encoding and passing on of genetic material. Amino acids are also fundamental in the building of muscle. There are twenty amino acids that the human body needs to function optimally. Our body can produce eleven important amino acids, but we need to obtain the other nine essential amino acids from eating protein, as our body is unable to make them. The greater amount of essential amino acids a protein has, the greater the quality of the protein. This is referred to as the biological value of protein. It is no surprise that animal tissue is more similar in a biochemical sense to human tissue than

COMBINING PLANT PROTEINS

Combining plant proteins enhances the biological value of protein that can be obtained from plant material. Corn, for example, is low in the essential amino acid lysine and hence has a low biological value, but it has a high amount of sulphur amino acids. Beans also have a low biological value because they have low amounts of sulphur amino acids but contain large amounts of lysine. If the two are combined, the total biological value of the protein is increased, as the deficiency in one is made up by the abundance in the other. This is why vegetarians are advised to combine plant proteins during any meal.

plant material. Red meat, fish and chicken, for example, contain all the essential amino acids, and therefore have a greater protein quality. Plant proteins have a short supply of at least one essential amino acid.

The 'protein quality' of any protein depends upon how many essential amino acids it has. If the protein has only six of the possible nine essential amino acids then it would have a low 'protein quality'. If, on the other hand, a protein had all nine essential amino acids, and they were enough to meet the human requirements, then this protein would be considered to have a high 'protein quality'.

A daily intake of 0.75 grams per kilogram of body weight is the approximate daily requirement of protein for inactive adults. For example, a 70-kilogram man would require 53 grams of protein per day, whereas a 95-kilogram man may require 71 grams per day. A 50-kilogram woman would require 40–50 grams of protein per day, and an 80-kilogram woman would need about 70 grams each day. The amount of protein required increases during periods of growth spurts, pregnancy and lactation. Active people, particularly those involved in intense weight training, also require a greater protein intake, approximately 1.2–1.7 grams per kilogram of body weight. This would be roughly 85 grams for a 70-kilogram man and 115 grams for a 95-kilogram man. On average, Australians (both men and women) eat too much protein each day – the average consumption is roughly 120 grams, and mainly in the form of red meat.

What happens to large intakes of protein?

Protein is continually broken down as well as produced in the body, but excess protein cannot be stored. The proteins produced in the body are hormones, enzymes, muscle tissue, and connective tissue such as elastin and collagen. On a daily basis there are about 250–300 grams of protein broken down and rebuilt in the body. This is termed 'protein turnover'. But of this 250–300 grams, the amount taken from eating is only around 90 grams. This essentially means that old proteins are broken down and replaced with newer proteins. Any excess protein is broken down and urinated out.

If proteins are consumed in large quantities, then the intake of carbohydrate and dietary fibre is reduced, as you can only eat a certain amount of food each day before you become full. The intake of fruits and vegetables is also limited in the diet to allow for larger protein intakes. In this case, the body is missing out on essential vitamins and minerals as well as high-fibre carbohydrates. There must be an appropriate balance of all these foods in the daily diet in order to meet all the body's energy needs. We already know that low intake of high-fibre carbohydrates can increase the risk of colon cancer and heart disease, and cells need the vitamins and minerals from fruit and vegetables to function optimally.

Be aware that if you are following a high-protein diet, there are often accompanying fats, such as a hamburger with cheese, pan-fried fish, steak and chips, and fatty lamb chops. It may be the case that while you think you are being healthy by eating lots of protein, you are consuming lots of fat at the same time. Make sure that your lamb chops are lean and that your fish is steamed, baked, grilled or only lightly fried in olive oil. Be aware also that contrary to many recently published theories, diets high in protein do increase the amount of insulin that is present in the blood (see page 62).

The dangers of a high-protein diet

When glucose is scarce in the body, as a result of following a diet high in protein and low in carbohydrate, the body is forced to use fatty acids (and protein) as an energy source. The breakdown of fatty acids results in a large amount of ketone bodies being produced, more in fact than the body can use. Ketone bodies are the leftover products after fats and proteins are broken down in the liver. Surplus ketone bodies can be quite dangerous, as they travel around in the blood, making it more acidic. This is a hazardous situation, as the increased acidic environment affects the ability of oxygen to be carried around in the blood. This could lead to a decreased amount of oxygen being delivered to the cells of the body. If cells are deprived of oxygen, then they ultimately die. An oversupply of ketone bodies can result in bad breath as well as dehydration.

Producing glucose from protein

When the carbohydrate intake is insufficient and glucose levels in the body are too low, the body can devour its own protein to produce glucose. This process is known as gluconeogenesis and occurs if you have eaten too much protein and not enough carbohydrate. In the breakdown of protein to form glucose, ammonia is produced. This is chemically identical to the ammonia contained in cleaning agents, but it is not harmful to the body as it is converted in the liver to a less toxic substance called urea, which is urinated out.

A high-protein diet results in muscle loss, as the body devours its own muscle, where protein is contained, in order to make glucose. A decrease in muscle mass will do nothing to enhance or promote fat loss or the loss of cellulite. The primary area where fat is used up, or burnt, is in the muscle, therefore a loss of lean muscle will slow down your metabolism and hinder fat loss. If your body is losing muscle, then you will have fewer muscle sites to burn up fat. While you may be pleased with the weight loss, you have not actually lost any fat and your body is not any healthier. A high-protein diet may also result in an increased calcium loss.

High-protein dieters beware; when protein is being broken down to be used as glucose, the production of enzymes, hormones, connective tissue, and hair and nails also dramatically decreases. This can lead to a body that doesn't function at an optimal level. Many of my female clients found that the texture, colour and strength of their skin, hair and nails improved dramatically by decreasing their protein intake and increasing their carbohydrate intake. Although you may be advised to eat vast amounts of protein with high biological values (good-quality proteins), once these proteins undergo gluconeogenesis, their biological value is drastically reduced. Hence the effectiveness of these proteins is diminished.

Food combining

Food combining is one of the great unfounded theories of this age. At one time it was thought that eating carbohydrates and proteins separately was much better for our nutrition and weight loss. One theory was that the enzymes responsible for the breakdown of proteins didn't function when the enzymes for carbohydrates did. On the contrary, the body can digest carbohydrates, proteins and fats simultaneously. The simple fact that our bodies can break down a peanut is ample evidence of this, as a peanut is made up of carbohydrate, fat and protein.

It has also been suggested that you shouldn't eat carbohydrates after 6 p.m., only proteins. Some athletes say that you should eat only protein after 6 p.m. because carbohydrates will just sit in your intestine or turn to fat. Protein, on the other hand, will be metabolised very quickly, they believe. In fact, it is the other way around. Carbohydrates are broken down roughly two hours after they are eaten and then converted and stored as glycogen, not fat. Protein, however, will sit in your stomach for many more hours, as amino acid metabolism is slow.

Amino acid supplements

Thirty minutes after eating a meal that includes about 100 grams of red meat, there is an increased uptake of branch chain amino acids into the muscles for use. A meal such as this would contain approximately 5 grams of branch chain amino acids, and only 1–2 grams would pass into the bloodstream per hour. Protein stays in your stomach for a long period of time and the absorption of amino acids is a slow process.

> ## BRANCH CHAIN AMINO ACIDS
> There is a lot of hype about branch chain amino acids, which are promoted and sold (expensively) as supplementary proteins necessary for the body. Yet they are found in sufficient quantities in everyday foods, including wholemeal bread, eggs, steak, low-fat yoghurt and skim milk. The amino acids leucine, isoleucine and valine are different from other amino acids in that they are broken down exclusively in muscle cells. They also make up one-third of muscle protein.

Supplementing the everyday diet with protein powders, and in particular amino acid supplements, boomed during the 1980s. It was thought that if the amino acids found in food promote muscle growth, then by adding amino acid supplements to the diet muscle mass would improve. However, there is no scientific evidence that amino acid powders help increase muscle mass or for that matter aid with recovery during and after extended physical activity. Although some strength-training athletes, quoting various studies, are convinced that these products work, these studies can be flawed in either method or interpretation. Research on this topic continues.

SUMMARY:

- carbohydrates should contribute about 60 per cent of the energy in our diet
- glucose is the preferred fuel for the brain and nervous system
- a diet high in complex carbohydrates can help you lose weight
- meals that are high in complex carbohydrates tend to fill you up more than meals that are high in fat
- your recommended protein intake should be about 20–25 per cent of your total daily intake
- high-protein diets that are low in carbohydrate can be detrimental to your health

SUGAR –
IS IT FATTENING?

Key messages for this chapter

YOU WILL DISCOVER:

- the conversion of sugar to fat is not the preferred pathway of the human metabolism
- sugars (which are carbohydrates) are stored as fat ONLY when we eat them in excessive amounts
- the main focus of our eating should be on cutting out fat, not cutting down on sugar/carbohydrates
- carbohydrates have been given a bad name by some unfounded theories and this chapter puts carbohydrates/sugar back on the winners list

The common questions (and their answers)

People are always concerned that sugar may be fattening. Apart from the question of 'how do you get rid of cellulite?' the next most frequently asked question is 'is sugar fattening?' This topic has been extensively discussed and exploited by many authors in their bid to make an impact on readers. Unfortunately sugar (remember that sugars are carbohydrates) and carbohydrates in general get a bad rap from:

- poorly researched diet books
- fad/popular magazines
- New Age theories with little scientific basis
- misleading advertising
- companies with a vested interest in their own weight-loss products
- some scientists who quote only studies that are done on animals

The relationship between sugar and fat is quite a remarkable one. Can a person who has a diet that is high in carbohydrates, such as bread, cereals, pasta and rice, put on fat? Does the body convert sugar to fat? Some people might argue that this process of converting sugar to fat is found in nature. Animals have been converting sugar to fat for thousands of years. Bees, for example, can convert honey (sugar) to wax (fat). Pigs can be fattened up on a diet of grains alone. But before jumping to the conclusion that our bodies function like those of bees or pigs we need to consider why humans are different with respect to these processes. It has been found that the enzymes responsible for the conversion of sugar to fat exist in much larger quantities in animals than they do in humans. It is therefore difficult to compare animals, insects and humans on this basis. In fact, even when sugar is consumed with large amounts of fat, such as in chocolate, cakes and biscuits, the sugar is converted immediately to glucose and used by the body. It is only the fat component of these foods that is stored as fat.

Sugars are carbohydrates.

As you learned in Chapter 2, the body can store relatively large amounts of carbohydrate as glycogen. These stores can be emptied quickly and hence need to be frequently topped up. In most fitness work done above half pace, for example, these carbohydrate stores can be quickly depleted.

Converting carbohydrates to fat

The process of the conversion of carbohydrates to fat is called de novo lipogenesis. For years this process seemed mysterious. However, scientists have now found that this process of converting sugar or carbohydrate to fat does exist but only in extreme cases such as the Gura Walla ritual. In a study during the 1990s of a traditional Cameroon bulking-up ritual, it was found that the Guru Walla tribes deliberately overfeed adolescent boys. These young men are forced to eat huge amounts of food, of which 70 per cent is carbohydrate, and the amount of carbohydrate intake is greater than the total amount of energy these adolescents use up during the day. They eat roughly 29 400 kJ of food per day, which is three times the amount of food consumed by the average Australian male, who eats roughly 11 000 kJ of food per day. Even elite cyclists on the Tour De France cycling race eat roughly only 24 000 kJ, and they cycle for the entire day, every day, for three weeks, covering 4000 kilometres. This, then, really is a case of severe overeating for the young tribesmen. The amount of energy they receive from carbohydrates is the same as eating eighty-six potatoes per day, and they also consume protein, to the equivalent of sixteen chicken breasts. Their fat intake is only 66 grams of fat per day and yet, remarkably, in ten weeks they put on only 133 grams of fat per day. This is less than 1 kilogram per week. From eating the equivalent of nearly 600 potatoes per week (6000 in ten weeks), not to mention the equivalent of 112 chicken breasts per week in protein, the amount of fat put on was quite small.

This study confirms that during severe, involuntary overeating, which is not the same as when we overindulge in junk food, the body can convert carbohydrate to fat. When we think about the concept of overeating, we very rarely overeat or 'pig-out' on good food. When was the last time you stuffed yourself at a dinner party on baked fish, pumpkin and roast potatoes? Can you recall a time that you have lost control and overeaten porridge? Most of the time when we overeat, we do so with junk food, party food and dining out, and it is our choice.

More recent studies show that single meals containing as much as 500 grams of carbohydrate produced no fat storage, but rather glycogen storage. This suggests that as long as the carbohydrate intake doesn't exceed the total amount of energy you expend each day, then carbohydrate will not be converted to fat. For example, if a woman expends her energy during a typical day doing various tasks such as travelling to and from work, being up and about for most of the day, helping to prepare dinner and then sleeping at night for six to seven hours, she uses around 9000 kJ of energy. This 9000 kJ translates roughly to 500 grams of carbohydrate. As long as she doesn't eat more than 500 grams of carbohydrate, then she will not significantly store carbohydrate fat.

Several other studies have been carried out to determine exactly how much carbohydrate we can eat before it is stored as fat. It has been shown that in cases of massive overfeeding of 1500 grams of carbohydrate, some fat storage began only after three days. From this study it is thought that once 700–1000 grams of carbohydrate is exceeded, carbohydrates are converted into fat tissue. Using advanced technology, studies show that the conversion of carbohydrate to fat is not the main fate of carbohydrates in the average Western diet. In one study, people who were confined to a metabolic ward consumed close to 18 900 kJ per day. Remember that the average Australian male consumes about 11 000 kJ per day. Of this 18 900, roughly 700 grams was from carbohydrate. This is about the equivalent of forty-eight medium-sized potatoes. They ate this way for seven to fourteen days. The amount of fat gained from the conversion of carbohydrate to fat was less than 1 gram of fat per day. As previously mentioned, the surplus carbohydrate was used in normal everyday activity, as well as being used to fill up the liver and muscle cells with glycogen.

> ## A HIGH-CARBOHYDRATE INTAKE MEANS
> - decreased fat intake
> - decreased amount of fat being stored
> - an increase in the amount of energy your body expends to convert carbohydrates to storage glycogen
> - an increased amount of carbohydrate usage
> - weight loss
> - body fat loss
> - although there is a decrease in fat use, your body will still burn significant amounts of fat

The conversion of carbohydrate to fat is an expensive process and costs the body a lot of energy. In fact, if we return to our analogy of storage costs, converting carbohydrate to fat costs 28 per cent of the total energy of the carbohydrate. If three large-sized potatoes were eaten (50 grams of carbohydrate) after many other carbohydrate dishes, then 28 per cent, or 14 grams, would be used to convert this to fat. That would leave only 36 grams stored as fat. Remember also that the storage of fat as fat is a very efficient process and only costs about 3 per cent.

It has always been assumed that excess carbohydrate is stored as fat. This is not the case. The conversion of sugar to fat is not the preferred pathway in humans. This is true for people on a typical Western diet, which consists of 35–45 per cent fat. Excess carbohydrate has other functions, such as being used as energy by the body. It is only when the carbohydrate intake exceeds a certain level, more than 550 grams per day, that carbohydrate is converted and stored as fat. Carbohydrate will primarily be converted into glucose and used as fuel for the moving muscles, to top up liver and muscle glycogen stores, and for other bodily functions.

You may say that if more carbohydrate than fat is used up in normal everyday activity, then wouldn't that mean that you would use less fat and hence put on weight? This is highly unlikely because you would actually be storing much less fat by eating a high-carbohydrate diet with reduced fat intake. If you reduced the amount of fat you ate by only 25 grams every day, then you could reduce the amount of fat stored on your body by as much as 170 grams per week or nearly 9 kilograms of fat per year.

The main focus of this book is to reduce the amount of fat that is easily stored as fat in our diet. If eating too many carbohydrates is your only problem, then you are most unlikely to have a problem losing fat. In what we have looked at so far, there are no adverse effects in following a diet that is normally high in carbohydrates.

I am not advocating that you eat copious amounts of sugar just because sugar isn't fattening. This is not the message. Sugary foods are fine as long as they are eaten in moderation. They shouldn't take the place of fibre-rich carbohydrates, and fruit and vegetables that provide essential vitamins and minerals and energy.

If I eat too much sugar, will I become a diabetic?

There is a fallacy that if you have too much glucose in your blood, and hence insulin, you will develop diabetes or 'insulin resistance'. There is no evidence that sugar or carbohydrates are involved in the development of diabetes. As a matter of fact, it has been medically shown that a diet high in complex carbohydrates can control and improve glucose tolerance.

Let the facts speak for themselves. In countries where people traditionally eat plenty of carbohydrates, the incidence of diabetes is quite low. There have been suggestions that sucrose, or table sugar, can be related to type 2 diabetes, because it produces higher levels of blood glucose when it is digested, and hence it may affect the release of insulin. In fact, due to the fact that sucrose contains a smaller sugar unit called fructose, the consumption of sucrose produces a smaller rise in blood glucose and insulin than the consumption of glucose or starch.

The main point is that if you are not a diabetic, then you won't get diabetes by eating sugar or carbohydrates, especially if your diet is balanced and you are active. Diabetes is hereditary or may occur if you become extremely overweight. If your insulin levels are raised, this is a natural response to what you are eating. Insulin levels are raised not only by carbohydrate, but by the intake of fat and protein as well. This is how the body functions normally so there is no need to fight this natural process.

SUMMARY:

- the conversion of sugar/carbohydrates to fat during normal healthy eating is highly unlikely
- sugars (which are carbohydrates) are likely to be stored as fat ONLY when we eat them in excessive amounts
- in our diet we should focus on cutting out fat, not cutting down on sugar/carbohydrates
- the best scientific studies show that high-carbohydrate diets do not lead to fat gain as described in some diet books
- you cannot develop diabetes by eating too much sugar

HOW THE BODY USES FAT

Key messages for this chapter

YOU WILL DISCOVER:

- how fat is treated by the body
- at what times fat is used as a fuel and at what times
  it is stored
- how the processes of releasing fat from the fat cell (lipolysis)
  and fat burning (oxidation) work
- insulin packs fat into fat cells
- insulin packs glucose into the liver and muscle cells
- insulin is raised by both carbohydrate and protein

Fat in the body

The process of fat stripping is complex and powerful. The average human being has enough stored fat to walk 800–2400 kilometres. If we were to walk continuously, then we could travel for eleven days with this energy supply. The process of removing fat from the fat cells, transporting this fat to the exercising muscles, then burning this fat as fuel functions like a finely tuned machine. There are several important points that must be considered when we try to understand this process.

Firstly, to transport fat out of the fat cell, the body must meet specific conditions. Ideal conditions are generally when we are resting, at least two hours after we have eaten, or during low-intensity activity. It also means that what you eat and when you eat will have an important bearing on the initial process of transporting fat out of the fat cell.

The next phase of fat stripping involves getting fat into the muscle cell where it can be burnt or 'used up' during periods of rest, light normal activity and exercise. Once again certain conditions must exist for this to happen. Fat moves out of fat cells relatively slowly, and hence it takes a while before you begin to use significant amounts. This process also depends upon the type of food you have eaten, when you eat, and what type of exercise you do.

The story of insulin completes the triad of fat-stripping mechanisms. Insulin regulates the levels of glucose in the blood and has been touted by many authors as being the main reason why we put on weight. However, as you will see, insulin is a normal and essential part of how our bodies deal with fat.

When do we use fat?

Let's have a look at how we use fat in our body during a normal day. We will do this by looking at a woman; let's call her Joanne. When Joanne wakes up in the morning the glucose levels in her blood, liver and muscles are low. Her body has spent roughly 1700 kJ of energy during sleep on all the bodily processes that make up her 'metabolism' (see page 4).

Along with glucose, her body has spent significant amounts of fat to keep these processes going. By eating a breakfast of some cereal and milk, Joanne replenishes some of the energy stores that she used up the night before, especially her glycogen stores. This is why eating a large breakfast can be extremely beneficial and why breakfast is considered by nutritionists to be the most important meal of the day. After a few hours, however, she is hungry again. Her storage of glucose is running low. This will need to be topped up and her hunger cravings signal this. Let's now take an even closer look at what happens to Joanne's energy stores and how her lunch affects these stores.

Joanne eats a couple of sandwiches with salad and salmon, a fruit juice, a small apple and a Turkish Delight chocolate bar. We will only consider the fate of the carbohydrates and the fat of Joanne's meal, as the protein is used by the body for repair and maintenance of tissues. We find that 65 per cent of her meal was carbohydrate, 10 per cent was fat, and 25 per cent was protein. Macronutrients, which are the main nutrients derived from eating carbohydrates, protein and fat, enter the blood, but only after they have been broken down to smaller molecules. Fat remains as fat, while all carbohydrates are converted to glucose after digestion.

Glucose is the body's major energy source just after a meal.

For the next thirty to sixty minutes the blood is like a carnival of activity, with high levels of glucose and fat being transported to their various destinations. The glucose enters the blood well before the creamy fat, which is absorbed firstly into the lymph system. Straight after a meal there is an abundance of glucose in the blood. There is even too much! This high level of glucose needs to be reduced so it is quickly converted and stored as glycogen or used immediately as fuel for the body. Therefore glucose is the dominant source of energy straight after a meal. Some of the glucose is stored in the liver cells (where roughly 70 grams can be stored), and in the muscle cells (where 400–500 grams can be stored). A fraction of glucose enters the other cells of the body such as the brain and heart where it can be burnt as fuel. Insulin responds to the body's demand for glucose by 'punching holes' in the muscle cells for fast storage of glucose as glycogen. The carnival of activity subsides within two to three hours, during which time the glucose has been stored.

Straight after a meal, the fate of fat is very different from that of carbohydrate. Fat is absorbed first into the lymph system, and then into the bloodstream. There isn't a 'hero's welcome' for fat as it is whisked away in the bloodstream. Fats are transported in the blood to the liver where they can be dispatched to the adipose tissue and stored as fat. It is not the dominant source of energy, and doesn't contribute significantly as a source of fuel so it is humbly stored (97 per cent of fat is stored). This storage of fat is rapid, and the fat cells take in fat like a sponge soaking up water. This paints a clear picture that shows fat is not used as a predominant source of fuel straight after a meal.

Insulin: the controller

In order for this hectic activity to be straightened out, the glucose and fat need to be under the orders of a strong 'foreman'. In this case the foreman is insulin. Insulin is a powerful hormone responsible for regulating the levels of glucose in the blood, and it 'punches holes' in the muscle cells to promote speedy storage of glucose as glycogen. This process is essential for any healthy, functioning body. At the same time, insulin also enhances fat storage. This is why when insulin is present, glucose is packed into liver and muscle cells and stored, and fat is packed into fat cells for storage. Insulin has other roles in the body, such as transporting amino acids to cells.

Just after eating a high-carbohydrate meal, glucose is in abundance and must be cleared from the blood, which takes two to three hours. This process is carried out mainly by insulin. As glucose in the blood increases, insulin is released. The more glucose there is, the more insulin is present. After approximately two to three hours, however, the amount of insulin in the blood decreases as most of the glucose has been mobilised into the body's cells. Even if the meal were high in fat, glucose would still be the dominant source of fuel immediately after the meal, but the time that it would take to clear the glucose would be less. Fat would then be called on to contribute to the body's energy demand. (In fact, if you could see the colour of the blood plasma after a high-fat meal, you would see a constant flow of a cream-like substance. This is the fat being transported to the liver or storage area.)

It must be stressed that when you eat a meal that is high in fat or protein, insulin is still released into the bloodstream. It is not just carbohydrates that raise insulin levels. This is the relationship between insulin and fat. In the next chapter you will discover how to use this relationship to your advantage.

Prime time for fat-stripping

As the amount of glucose that the body can store is limited and can be depleted very quickly, there simply isn't enough stored glucose to meet the demands of the brain and nervous system, and the other energy needs of the body for a sustained period of time. Some time after a meal, when all the glucose from the meal has been stored, and no more is being absorbed from the intestine, the body must ration the use of glucose, only delivering small amounts of glucose to the brain and nervous system, where it is vital for function. At this stage the body decreases the use of glucose by all other organs. However, these other organs still require a source of energy in order for them to keep functioning. As most of the glucose in the blood is finally cleared, the body needs to find an alternate source of energy. At the end of the two to three-hour period after a meal, the glucose and insulin levels are low, and hence there isn't sufficient insulin to stop fats from being released into the bloodstream. Fat now becomes the dominant source of energy used by the body.

Large amounts of fat can be burnt as fuel two to three hours after a meal.

This system is sometimes referred to as 'glucose sparring'. The body is able to do this with the help of the hormone glucagon. Glucagon has the inverse role of insulin in the body. When the body requires energy, glucagon signals to the liver to release glucose into the blood and to the adipose tissue to release fat into the blood. Therefore two to three hours after a meal, the conditions in the body are ideal for fat stripping.

Removing fat from the fat cell

Lipolysis is the term used to describe the removal of fat from the fat-storage cells. Fat is stored in storage sites around the body, called adipose tissue or fat cells. When fat is eaten, only

3 per cent of it is used in digesting, breaking it down, transporting and storing it (see page 27). For example, if you ate a 50-gram block of cheese, which may contain 12 grams of fat, then you would store 11 grams. It costs the body a minimal amount of energy to store fat.

It is easy for the body to store fat, but very difficult to remove it from the fat cells.

To transport this fat out of the cell, however, is not as easy as putting it there in the first place. Remember that to date there are no natural products that can burn fat, or for that matter remove fat from its fat cell. To get fat out of its fat cell it needs a kick-start. Exercise can provide this start by activating the hormone called adrenaline (also called epinephrine). Stress has almost the same effect. Adrenaline binds to the fat cells and activates fat-breaking enzymes, which in turn allow fat to leave the storage cells and ooze out into the blood. This process gets 'kicked' into action in the two to three hours after a meal. As fat oozes out of the fat cells, it doesn't move rapidly: it takes some time before it can be used as an energy source. These fats are released as individual units called free-fatty acids (or FFAs). Once in the bloodstream, FFAs are transported to be used as fuel. At this stage the hormone glucagon not only stimulates the release of FFAs into the bloodstream, but also stops the release of glucose into the bloodstream.

This is why exercise should be done two to three hours after your last meal. It takes that long before fat can be burnt as fuel. Fitness instructors advise their clients to be active for longer than 15 minutes to give the body a chance to move fat out of the storage areas and into working muscles. This process of lipolysis also works best during low-intensity exercise such as walking when adrenaline is increased.

Burning fat

Once fats are released into the blood by the process of lipolysis they are transported to the site where they are needed as a source of energy. Muscle cells, for example, can use huge amounts of fat for energy but it is hard to get large amounts of fat into these cells at once as this process is quite slow. Fat moves slowly into the cells, as it must cross the cell membrane, and then it must be transported into the furnace called the mitochondria, where, like a piece of wood, it will provide energy for the muscle. Fats are carried into the furnace with the help of a substance called carnitine (also known as CAT). This process of burning fat is called fat oxidation.

Like lipolysis, the oxidation of fat is limited to certain circumstances. When there is an abundance of fat being released into the bloodstream (lipolysis), then more fat can be taken up and burnt (oxidation). But when the release of fat into the bloodstream is hindered, such as when there are high levels of insulin in the blood, then there is less fat available to be taken into the body cells and used. Straight after a meal both lipolysis and oxidation are decreased, as insulin is present. A lack of oxygen, in instances of running fast or lifting heavy equipment, also decreases lipolysis and hence oxidation, as fats need oxygen to move around the body and to be burnt in the cells. Walking at a good pace and light jogging can dramatically increase both the release of fat and its use as energy.

SPORTS AMENORRHEA

This condition is defined as a change or complete loss of menstrual function. It commonly occurs in women who exercise frequently and eat relatively small amounts. The danger of this is a reduction in oestrogen levels. Chronically low oestrogen levels are linked with loss of bone density, and hence 'osteoporosis'.

If the process of fat oxidation is used to its fullest, then a person's body can take more fat into the fat cells and use more fat as fuel.

Not eating: the classic scenario for weight loss?
One of the most tried and failed methods for losing weight and fat is just not eating or eating very small amounts – if you don't eat, then how can you put on weight, right? In theory it makes

sense that if you eat little food and expend a lot of energy, then you must lose weight. Actually, you can do serious damage to your body by not eating. Let's explore the problems and their impact on the body.

Firstly, we know that the body, particularly the brain, needs glucose to function. If you are not eating sufficient amounts of food, where does the body find glucose and other forms of energy? The body finds this glucose by breaking down protein, which makes up much of the body's muscle mass. A major source of protein in the body is muscle. By breaking down muscle large amounts of amino acids are delivered to the liver where they can be converted to glucose (see pages 34–5). This muscle loss will register on the scales as a decreased body weight. You may be delighted, as your diet seems to be working.

However, this decrease in muscle actually has a detrimental effect on the body's ability to lose weight. This is because the more muscle mass you have, the higher your metabolism. Remember metabolism is the energy the body spends on digesting, breaking down, transporting and storing food, as well as the energy needed to keep your heart beating, your lungs functioning, your kidneys filtering and your brain thinking. The greater the muscle mass, then the greater the amount of energy your muscles need to be supplied with to carry out all these functions properly. Hence when a person eats sparsely, the body still tries to maintain fat storage in case of even leaner times ahead, so it is not fat but protein that is sacrificed to keep the metabolism functioning. This is no way to lose cellulite or fat.

Many low-energy diets or periods of not eating will eventuate in muscle loss. Over a period of time, muscle loss means that your body and skin condition will deteriorate. The amount of water in your cells decreases, not to mention being irritable, having bad breath, headaches and a lack of concentration. Be aware that any diet promising to help you 'lose 10 kilograms in 10 days' or 'drop three dress sizes in three weeks' means a loss of valuable lean muscle, as lean muscle can supply the necessary energy much quicker than body fat. Inadequate nutrition such as insufficient iron, calcium, protein and vitamins are other negative outcomes of not eating or following low-energy diets. You can be sure, too, that any weight that you lose on a quick-fix fad diet will be put back on in 99 per cent of cases.

Does your body burn more fat if you eat more fat?

This is an interesting question, as we have clearly established in Chapter 3 that if you eat more carbohydrates, then your body burns more carbohydrates. Unfortunately eating more high-fat food will not cause your body to burn more fat. The current scientific research tells us that any excess fat consumed is just stored. Even with a rather fast metabolism your body can only use a certain amount of fat. It must also be noted that obese and post-obese people do not increase the amount of fat they burn by eating large amounts of fat. This excess of fat is stored as fat.

What about following a high-protein diet?

In this chapter we have seen that when we eat carbohydrates, such as bread, cereal, pasta and potatoes, insulin levels in the body are raised, shutting down fat usage for a short period of time. This is the human body's normal response to a carbohydrate intake. This necessary and normal physiological function of a healthy body has unfortunately been exploited and abused by so-called 'fat-loss experts'. These so-called experts claim that in order to avoid raising insulin levels (having no insulin in the blood will enhance fat usage), you should cut down on carbohydrates, or cut them out altogether. They claim that you should replace them with plenty of protein.

Protein and insulin

The effect of protein on insulin levels is one of the most controversial points in human physiology today. Most of us understand the relationship between carbohydrates and insulin, but we very rarely hear about the relationship between protein and insulin. This relationship has been conveniently left out of most diet books as it confounds many modern-day theories about weight loss. When we eat carbohydrates, glucose in the blood increases, and so insulin levels in the blood are also raised (see pages 53–4). When insulin is present, the amount of fat being used by the body decreases. What is not so well known outside scientific circles is that when protein is eaten, insulin is released into the blood stream. This is a physiological fact and a perfectly normal function of a healthy body. Any person studying biochemistry or advanced nutrition can verify this.

At the Department of Biochemistry, Human Nutrition Unit, at the University of Sydney, Dr Susanne Holt and her team lead the world in the field of how insulin works in the body. Dr Holt and her team have looked at how much insulin protein produces as compared to fats and carbohydrates. They measured the insulin produced by eating equal energy amounts (1000 kJ) of pasta, rice, cheese, fish, and beef at different times.

INSULIN PRODUCED IN THE BLOOD (pmol.min/L)

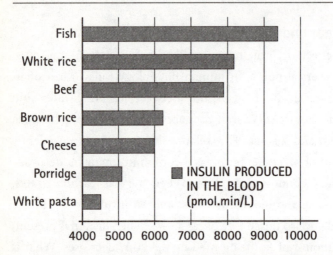

These results show that protein increases insulin levels in the blood as much as, if not more than, carbohydrates. As you can see, cheese, which is fat, produces a greater amount of insulin than white pasta, which is a carbohydrate. Fish, a protein, produces more than twice as much insulin as white pasta, and so on. Remember, once insulin is present in the blood the amount of fat being used by the body decreases. So proteins and fats as well as carbohydrates can suppress the use of fat by the body.

SUMMARY:
- fat is used at different times during the day by the body
- when glucose is abundant in the bloodstream, fat is stored, or present in very small amounts
- glucose is abundant in the blood after a meal
- Two to three hours after eating, when blood glucose is low, fat becomes the predominant source of fuel
- lipolysis is the process where fat is released from the adipose tissue into the bloodstream
- oxidation is the process of burning fat as a source of energy
- eating protein and carbohydrate can halt fat usage for a short period of time

THE ENERGY COST OF FOOD

Key messages for this chapter

YOU WILL DISCOVER:
- how easy it is to consume large amounts of fat
- how planning and preparation can minimise the amount of fat you eat
- how to use the Bilsborough Fat Cost Chart
- the real costs of eating too much fat
- how fat and exercise are linked
- that even though you have had a bad day, you can make up for it tomorrow

The years catching up with you

When most of us were younger we didn't really have to worry about fat. This is especially true for those of us who were involved in some form of activity, whether it were football, jazz ballet, walking to school and back, or just getting down to the beach for a swim. In what many people refer to as 'the good old days', this higher level of physical activity kept fat off our bodies. It seemed that we could live on junk food, skip meals and have a hectic schedule, and the kilos just never accumulated. Then one day, from absolutely nowhere, came the belly or the bottom from hell. This is very common for most sportspeople who have an active lifestyle and then suddenly stop. This may also be true for people who have never had a fat problem and then one day, BANG, there it is.

In this chapter we will look at the lifestyles of typical people and see how they can mend their ways and regain the figures of their youth!

Off to a bad start

John's done the right thing for the first time in a long time. He has actually made breakfast. Into an oily pan he tosses a handful of bacon pieces with a couple of eggs. He slaps this onto two pieces of toast, and the taste is, he feels, well worth the effort. As he races for the train he justifies his bacon and egg splurge by telling himself that at least he has done the right thing and had breakfast. *John's made a bad start!* Let's follow his eating pattern throughout the day.

The bacon and oil contain 31 grams of fat. Now this may not mean much to the average person, but the Fat-Stripping Diet converts this to a value that you can understand. The bacon and eggs could *potentially* take around 85 minutes to walk off, which is equivalent to walking a distance of around 9 kilometres. If you had the motivation and ability then you could try some light jogging for 71 minutes for a distance of 10.2 kilometres. These values for walking are taken from the Bilsborough Fat Cost Chart (see pages 162–5). We will focus on walking in this book, but will include how much time and how far you need to travel during a light jog for those who do like jogging.

Midmorning slowly arrives, and John takes a much-needed coffee break with a few of his co-workers. He only intended to buy a coffee and then get straight back into work, as it is a busy day, but he gets held up, engrossed in conversation. He feels a little peckish, so he grabs an iced doughnut. The iced doughnut contains 19 grams of fat and *potentially* requires 55 minutes of walking, which is equivalent to a distance of roughly 5.7 kilometres. Once again, to physically run this food off during a light jog would take 47 minutes and a distance of 7 kilometres.

Lunchtime finally arrives and John is famished. Someone suggests a tasty cheap restaurant around the corner, and he hastily agrees. Looking for something reasonably healthy, he opts for some baked chicken breast, with avocado and a light salad without any dressing. It might have been better to buy a sandwich, or a roll, but he is famished, and didn't think that *just* a roll would fill him up. The decision may have cost John – to the tune of 26 grams of fat, as avocados are quite fattening. Once again the time and distance needed to burn this fat is high. In fact, he would need to walk for 75 minutes, covering 7.8 kilometres. If he were to jog then this would convert to running 8.7 kilometres in a time of 61 minutes. Cream and oil used to make the light sauce that covered the chicken also contained 14 grams of fat. This amounts to 46 minutes of walking, covering a distance of 4.7 kilometres, or light jogging for 37 minutes covering 5.4 kilometres. John's learning fast, however, and the bottom line is that he's just having a bad day.

No bad day is ever so detrimental that it cannot be fixed in the following days. He may have the notion to do the right thing, but like most people, including myself, circumstances and situations sometimes get the better of us. This is compounded especially when we have no understanding of what the cost of eating a diet that is high in fat really means. So far John has made it through lunch, and he's now rather full, although there's a very small vanilla sponge cake beckoning to be eaten. A third of it remained on his plate, and he realises that he probably shouldn't have bought it. It's added a further 36 minutes, and 3.7 kilometres, to his ever-building fat bank. Understanding roughly how much fat, including hidden fat, is in foods is important for you to make better food choices.

The cost so far

The amount of energy that John will need to expend will depend upon how much fat he has eaten during the day. These amounts are shown in the table opposite. The total fat and activity level reached for the day is already quite high. This may seem surprising considering that John's eaten salad, avocado and chicken, rather than deep-fried fish, chips, and a cream cake. Unfortunately even the healthiest meal may contain hidden fats. This starts in the way a meal is cooked (whether it is fried in oil or baked), or the way it is presented (oil on the salad). All these hidden fats add up and it is up to you to take charge, and understand how to add up this total fat and its accompanying physical cost.

If is still isn't getting any better

John has worked quite late and arrives home just after 7.30 p.m. Some lamb chops have been defrosted from the morning so he places them under the grill rather than frying them. He chops up and stir-fries some vegetables, and adds a few slices of bread to his meal. Dinner is ready. With this meal, John would have added the following values to his fat bank: 42 grams of fat, and 104 minutes of walking covering 10.7 kilometres, or 92 minutes of running covering 13.2 kilometres. But before it's time to close the doors on his fat bank there's also the 'chocolate factor'. John may say, 'But they were only nine small squares!' They were small but very expensive in terms of his fat bank. Add another 12 grams of fat, with 41 minutes of walking covering 4.2 kilometres, or 34 minutes of running covering 4.8 kilometres. Let's see how John's day tallies.

JOHN'S DAY

	FAT (grams)	WALKING TIME (minutes)	WALKING DISTANCE (kilometres)	RUNNING TIME (minutes)	RUNNING DISTANCE (kilometres)
Breakfast	31	85	9	71	10
Morning snack	19	55	5.7	47	7
Lunch	40	121	12.5	98	14.1
Afternoon snack	9	36	3.7	28	4
Dinner	54	145	14.9	126	18
TOTAL	**153**	**442**	**45.8**	**370**	**53.1**

The real *potential* cost of fat, in terms of exercise, has not been clearly established in non-scientific publications. The Fat-Stripping Diet, however, clearly shows you that the more fat you eat, the more exercise you must perform to strip this fat off your body. John's daily consumption has shown that 153 grams of fat may require 442 minutes of walking and a distance of 45.8 kilometres. This fat consumption also translates to 370 minutes of jogging at a good pace, covering 53.1 kilometres.

The Fat-Stripping Diet does not advocate that you walk or jog these distances, even if you could. The idea here is to understand that if you eat fat then you will store most of it. Rather than walk for 442 minutes to burn off this fat, it is easier to just 'not eat it' in the first place. The tables in this chapter provide an understanding of the ballpark figure in terms of exercise. This means that for some men it might take 350 minutes of walking but for others it might only take 284 minutes. On the other hand it may take you 442 minutes. These values are average values. Before you start saying 'I'll never be able to lose fat now', take heart.

What must also be taken into account with respect to the entire day is the fact that between meals, during light activity and while you are sleeping, the human body relies on fat as a source of energy. The body can only use a certain amount of fat every day and the leftover fat, or fat surplus, can either be stored as fat or stripped during exercise. Two average values have been chosen as the fat surplus values. The latest research has been investigating what the minimal amount of fat is that the body needs to function at a healthy level. These values are 60 grams of fat for men and 41 grams of fat for women. Once you have eaten a greater amount of fat than this value in any day, you need to burn this off, or it will be stored as body fat. Remember that if you are carrying fat that you want to lose, then once you get your 12–17 grams of essential fatty acids (see pages 5–6), let the body use the remainder of fat from its own fat stores.

We can see that the 153 grams of fat has grossly exceeded our fat surplus values. John has breached this value by 93 grams (153 less 60). This means that the body will burn a maximum of approximately 60 grams of fat without John having to do any exercise. Anything left over must be *stripped* during exercise or stored as fat. Taking this into account our values in the table on page 69 can be scaled down to look a little less daunting (see below).

JOHN'S FAT BANK

FAT (grams)	WALKING TIME (minutes)	WALKING DISTANCE (kilometres)	RUNNING TIME (minutes)	RUNNING DISTANCE (kilometres)
93	230	20.8	190	24

The hard facts still remain, however, and if John cannot find the time to walk 20.8 kilometres, or run 24 kilometres, then he will store this fat on his body.

Total cost in the fat bank?
Remember that the situation can only get better. John's aim would be to have as little fat as possible in his fat bank, on as many days as possible. One bad day won't ruin your lifestyle. John had already exceeded the fat surplus limit of 60 grams of fat by lunchtime, so from then onwards all the fat he ate needed to be burnt off. If your fat bank looks like John's, then warning lights should start flashing. If your day-to-day eating habits are similar to John's, then this will be the key reason why you are not reducing weight or body fat. It will be the result of having given up walking with your neighbour in the morning, or stopped going to the gym, or even ceased to continue your own

exercise program. You may have previously blamed your exercise program for not being effective enough, but in fact not too many exercise programs would cater for this kind of fat intake. If you were a marathon runner or a triathlete, then you would probably do enough exercise for fat loss of this nature, but that's about it. The bottom line is that exercise programs are *generally* not flawed. It is not understanding the physical cost of what we eat that has so many implications, as you can now see. There are several good activities that can maximise your fat-loss potential (see pages 87–91).

One of the aims of *The Fat-Stripping Diet* is to help you understand that this cost of a high-fat diet is quite demanding, and even the most motivated person would have difficulty in exercising at this rate. As we have discussed before, this method of understanding the physical cost of fat can help explain why it is so easy to put on weight, and in particular, fat, and why it is so hard to remove. The scenario followed so far shows us that we may not clearly understand where the hidden fats lie. It is also common to feel at ease once we have eaten some vegetables or a salad, because we associate these foods with good eating. They are sometimes eaten, however, because we believe they may balance out the foods that are not so healthy. For example, we think the salad may balance out the doughnut. There is no such balance, and the foods high in fat mean that we maintain a fat surplus in our body. As a consumer, you need to now make some informed decisions.

What would happen for a woman?

We have previously discussed why women and men burn different amounts of energy. We will use this information to illustrate the differences in the amount of energy that Joanne would have to expend compared to John. We will also assume that the meal types are the same, only slightly smaller in size.

JOANNE'S DAY

	FAT (grams)	WALKING TIME (minutes)	WALKING DISTANCE (kilometres)	RUNNING TIME (minutes)	RUNNING DISTANCE (kilometres)
Breakfast	27	95	9.8	84	11.2
Morning snack	19	72	7.4	62	8.3
Lunch	33	126	13.1	112	14.8
Afternoon snack	7	36	4	30	4.7
Dinner	45	148	15.2	128	17.8
TOTAL	**131**	**477**	**49.5**	**416**	**56.7**

As this table clearly illustrates, Joanne has also had a bad start to her day. Although she has eaten smaller quantities than John, she has a slower metabolism than her male counterpart. This slower metabolism coupled with the high-fat intake means she not only has a mammoth amount of exercise to do, she has greatly exceeded her fat surplus limit of 41 grams. Remember this is the amount of fat her body will use during a day. For Joanne, there is a surplus of 90 grams of fat that needs to be stripped off (131 less 41).

Because she has exceeded her limit of 41 grams of fat, all her fat eaten after she has consumed 41 grams of fat must either be stripped off during exercise or stored as fat. The total surplus fat cost of her day's eating is shown in the table below. Remember once again that this book is not advocating that you do this amount of exercise, but rather making you aware that foods high in fat can take a long time to work off.

JOANNE'S FAT BANK

FAT (grams)	WALKING TIME (minutes)	WALKING DISTANCE (kilometres)	RUNNING TIME (minutes)	RUNNING DISTANCE (kilometres)
90	280	29.2	224	38

The silver lining

The first step towards a better eating plan is to replace high-fat foods with low-fat or no-fat options. Physical activity is *not* essential in order for the Fat-Stripping Diet to work, but it is important to keep your heart healthy and to maintain an adequate fitness level. After ten weeks on the diet you will see a significant reduction in body fat, but you may find that your fat stripping has reached a sticking point. At this stage you may need to include some kind of activity in your lifestyle to keep your body fat-free.

The better your food intake, the less work you need to do, and the less fat you need to strip from your body. Remember that the body has to work harder on the Fat-Stripping Diet to store carbohydrate as glycogen. You will also have only a small amount of fat coming in, which will be readily used by the body. Use the table of common and high-fat foods and their accompanying fat grams, walking and running distances and times (see pages 148–51) as a guide to help you choose foods that will reduce your exercise time. This process of adjusting your eating habits may take some time, so don't be disappointed if you don't stick to it every day. Remember, the more days that you eat less fat, the less fat you will have to strip. If you follow this part of the diet, then you should notice changes in your bodyweight in a very short period of time.

Once you've started on this program and begin to see initial changes, encourage yourself, congratulate yourself, and you will improve even further. All you need is a small spark of motivation to snowball into better results. Sometimes people underestimate small changes, and see them as insignificant. Nothing could be further from the truth. It is in fact these small changes that form cascading effects not only in terms of weight and fat loss, but also as motivational springboards.

Off to a good start

Let's start the day again, only this time with someone much wiser and much more prepared than John or Joanne. Let's follow Alex, and use his nutritional habits as a rough guide. Alex knows the physical cost of food (because he has read *The Fat-Stripping Diet*), and therefore is determined to minimise his high-fat foods in order to lose fat. He is on a mission! For breakfast Alex has breakfast cereal with low-fat milk, with a cup of coffee. He tends not to like breakfast, as he never feels hungry, so he eats quite a small meal. Keeping this in mind he is aware that at around midmorning he will be very hungry so he takes a low-fat muesli bar and a banana with him to work. This accompanies his usual 10 a.m. coffee. He has prepared two sandwiches for his lunch, ham and salad, but no cheese. He finishes off lunch with a diet soft drink and an apple.

So far, so good for Alex. In his fat bank Alex has accumulated just 5 grams of fat, which *potentially* converts to 24 minutes of walking covering 2.6 kilometres, or 20 minutes of running covering 2.8 kilometres. If we remember John, then the difference is very significant. Without some basic knowledge, 5 grams of fat could well mean 5 balls of string. People have struggled to understand exactly why these 5 grams of fat are not particularly beneficial to their bodies. Remember that John had by this time (lunchtime) *already* consumed 99 grams of fat, and had a surplus of 39 grams of fat. Alex, on the other hand, has only consumed 5 grams of fat, and his body will burn that up without Alex having to exercise at all. By watching his fat, Alex still has 55 grams of fat that he could eat if he wanted to.

When we take a close look at what Alex ate, the quality of food seems quite substantial and he hasn't starved or eaten 'bird seed', as some would put it. All he has done is simply prepared his food with the understanding of the physical cost of it. In the middle of the afternoon Alex has plenty of water crackers with some spicy salsa dip. This small meal was also pre-packed, and keeps his energy levels up until he gets home. His preparation has not only served the purpose of keeping him relatively hunger-free, but it has also served a second and more important purpose: it has stopped him from snacking on junk food. Sometimes when we feel like something light, we fall into the trap of purchasing doughnuts, ice cream, chocolates, or chips. If we snack on these foods on a continual basis, then the fat in our fat bank builds up. This situation can so easily be avoided if preparation is given a high priority.

ALEX'S DAY

	FAT (grams)	WALKING TIME (minutes)	WALKING DISTANCE (kilometres)	RUNNING TIME (minutes)	RUNNING DISTANCE (kilometres)
Breakfast	0.3	0	0	0	0
Morning snack	0.2	0	0	0	0
Lunch	5	24	2.6	20	2.8
Afternoon snack	0.1	0	0	0	0
Dinner	8	33	3.4	26	3.7
TOTAL	13.6	57	6	46	6.8

For dinner Alex prepares some baked snapper, with vegetables. This is served with some bread and a glass of white wine. For dessert Alex has a couple of scoops of low-fat ice cream and that concludes his eating for the day. In total his dinner added a further 8 grams of fat to his overall fat intake.

In terms of exercise Alex added 33 minutes of walking covering 3.4 kilometres, or 26 minutes of running covering 3.7 kilometres. This 8 grams of fat still leaves Alex within his 60-gram fat surplus range. In fact, Alex has actually lost almost 47 grams of fat today (60 − 13).

Once again, let's compare subjects. Alex's fat intake is 80 grams less than John's (see page 71), and he doesn't need to subtract 60 grams from his fat intake because he has not exceeded the fat-surplus point. If Alex was to exercise, however, he would undoubtedly lose more fat weight than if he was to simply burn off the fat he has just eaten through normal bodily processes. John may do some of the walking or running, but it would be highly unlikely that he would walk all 20.8 kilometres. Unless he started to plan his eating, fat would just continue to accumulate on a daily and weekly basis.

THE FAT BANK: ALEX VS JOHN

	FAT (grams)	WALKING TIME (minutes)	WALKING DISTANCE (kilometres)	RUNNING TIME (minutes)	RUNNING DISTANCE (kilometres)
John	93	230	20.8	190	24
Alex	13.6	0	0	0	0

Easy steps to success

Alex has shown that by having a good knowledge of the physical cost of food, and combining this with some simple preparation, he can not only eat very well, but he can feel quite full. There is still a need to perform some exercise as this will keep his heart healthy and help maintain a reasonable level of fitness. The list of foods that Alex can choose from is abundant, and he has banished the notion that a diet should be sparse, or one that contains just fruit and vegetables. In fact, Alex could have eaten more food if he'd wanted to, as long as the fat content was low. Remember that he had nearly 47 grams of fat to spare.

The three cases we have looked at so far cover the extremes. Two cases showed John and Joanne eating rather badly in terms of fat intake, while Alex ate incredibly well. Let's look at two people, a man and a woman, who eat what most of us would consider a normal diet. Rachel eats reasonably well through the day with occasional splurges.

For breakfast she has a bowl of muesli and a banana with a cup of coffee. Midmorning she eats an apple and two biscuits. For lunch she has a salad sandwich, a chocolate bar, fruit juice and a biscuit. She snacks on small piece of chocolate at about three o'clock. For dinner she has a small serve of lasagna and salad with some cheesecake and fruit salad for sweets.

On the surface Rachel's day seems to be rather good, although at a glance her only obvious pitfall is the chocolate bar and a standard small slice of cheesecake. 'You've got to have some fun,' I can hear many of my clients say! The total amount of fat that Rachel has eaten for the day is 66 grams. This isn't too much over our fat surplus value of 41 grams, but it is still over.

RACHEL'S DAY

	FAT (grams)	WALKING TIME (minutes)	WALKING DISTANCE (kilometres)	RUNNING TIME (minutes)	RUNNING DISTANCE (kilometres)
Breakfast	3	22	2.4	19	2.8
Morning snack	6	33	3.2	27	3.9
Lunch	16	61	7.3	54	8.1
Afternoon snack	10	45	4.8	38	5.7
Dinner	31	107	11.1	95	12.8
TOTAL	**66**	**268**	**28.8**	**233**	**33.3**

These figures become less daunting when we subtract 41 grams of fat, which the body will burn itself.

RACHEL'S FAT BANK

FAT (grams)	WALKING TIME (minutes)	WALKING DISTANCE (kilometres)	RUNNING TIME (minutes)	RUNNING DISTANCE (kilometres)
25	88	9.1	69	9.6

As the table indicates, the amount of activity needed to strip this fat from its fat cell is quite large, even though we thought that Rachel ate reasonably well. Although 25 grams is not a lot of fat to deposit, accumulation of small amounts of fat over weeks, months and years is a reason why we find ourselves with excess fat 'all of a sudden'. Rachel could make a big difference by simply cutting out the cheesecake and perhaps the biscuits at morning tea.

Brian follows a similar 'average' day. He starts with a large bowl of muesli and a banana with a cup of coffee. Mid-morning he eats an apple, two biscuits and a lamington. For lunch he has two salad sandwiches, a chocolate bar, fruit juice and a biscuit. He snacks on a small piece of chocolate at about three o'clock just like Rachel. For dinner he has a large serve of lasagna and salad with some cheesecake and fruit salad for sweets.

BRIAN'S DAY

	FAT (grams)	WALKING TIME (minutes)	WALKING DISTANCE (kilometres)	RUNNING TIME (minutes)	RUNNING DISTANCE (kilometres)
Breakfast	4	21	1.9	18	2.6
Morning snack	11	39	3.8	32	4.5
Lunch	20	60	5.5	49	7.1
Afternoon snack	10	38	3.4	30	4.2
Dinner	45	118	10.8	98	14.1
TOTAL	90	276	25.4	227	32.5

The large serving of lasagna (25 grams of fat) really hits the spot, and while the cheesecake (23 grams of fat) is a generous helping, it is still just the one slice. Like Rachel, Brian has eaten reasonably well with respect to his fat intake during the day. Although he ate a chocolate bar, biscuits, and some chocolate he totalled 45 grams of fat until he got home. Once again he hasn't eaten as well as Alex or as badly as John, he is just a bloke who thinks that he eats okay.

As we have done with all our clients in this chapter we have deducted the amount of fat that the body will use during the course of the day, in Brian's case 60 grams. This subtraction leaves Brian with an excess of 30 grams of fat for the day. He would need to walk for 82 minutes covering nearly 7.5 kilometres. Although 30 grams per day doesn't seem like an unmanageable amount, it could add up to 11 kilograms for the year (30 grams × 365 days in a year = 10.95 kilograms).

BRIAN'S FAT BANK

FAT (grams)	WALKING TIME (minutes)	WALKING DISTANCE (kilometres)	RUNNING TIME (minutes)	RUNNING DISTANCE (kilometres)
30	82	7.5	63	9.7

As you can see, small changes to our 'normal' eating can make a dramatic impact on the amount of fat that the body will store. The challenge for you is to maintain a healthy eating pattern that keeps inside your fat surplus point (60 grams for men and 41 grams for women). If you can achieve this, then you are well on the way to achieving fat loss, and consequently weight loss. The tables on pages 148–153 have been constructed to help you identify high-fat foods. They also have the respective times and distances for walking and running. As part of your first step in the Fat-Stripping Diet, it is important to roughly note down each day what foods you have eaten, and how much fat is contained in each of them. If these values exceed 60 grams for men, or 41 grams for women, you have a fat surplus. As demonstrated in the previous example, subtract 60 or 41 from your total fat and then use the tables to determine your physical cost.

High-fat fad diets

Without even knowing it, most of the Western population eats a high-fat diet. In fact, there are over 1 billion overweight people in the world. This is almost as many people as are starving or undernourished in the Third World. If you are concerned about your changing body shape and losing those extra kilograms, you should assess your diet to determine how much fat you are really consuming each day. You may be consuming more than you thought. People always say to me, 'If I'm using heaps of olive oil, which is good fat, then I can't get fat, right?' Wrong. Remember that an excess of even good fat is stored as fat. Fats that you cannot see, such as on your salad in your fried rice, continually add up as storage fat. The human body requires only a certain amount of fat for energy to function every day – any fat over that amount is stored in the body.

Everyone who has read this chapter always tells me how amazed they are that it takes so much time to work off body fat. It should make sense then that any book or any person advocating a diet high in fat or one that lets you eat as much fat as you like (even if it is good fat) must surely misunderstand the basic function of exercise metabolism. If, for example, you ate a diet that was 50, 60, 70 or 80 per cent fat, then this is how much fat an average man and woman would store each day.

MEN: THE COST OF HIGH-FAT DIETS

FAT IN DIET (grams)	WALKING TIME (minutes)	WALKING DISTANCE (kilometres)
50 per cent (145 – 60) = 85 grams	210	19
60 per cent (175 – 60) = 115 grams	284	25.7
70 per cent (203 – 60) = 143 grams	353	32
80 per cent (232 – 60) = 172 grams	425	38.4

WOMEN: THE COST OF HIGH-FAT DIETS

FAT IN DIET (grams)	WALKING TIME (minutes)	WALKING DISTANCE (kilometres)
50 per cent (105 – 41) = 64 grams	202	21
60 per cent (127 – 41) = 86 grams	258	28
70 per cent (148 – 41) = 107 grams	321	35
80 per cent (170 – 41) = 129 grams	387	42

SUMMARY:

- most of the time we consume large amounts of fat, without knowing it
- planning and preparation can minimise the amount of fat you eat, especially if you plan to have food with you during the times when you know you will be hungry
- the fat cost chart is a very effective method of understanding the real cost of fat
- the real cost of eating too much fat shows that fat is easy to put on but very difficult to get off
- remember that although you may have a bad day, you can make up for it tomorrow

FAT-STRIPPING EXERCISES

Key messages for this chapter

YOU WILL DISCOVER:
- the best exercises to lose fat are low-level intensity, such as fast walking, light jogging, or cycling
- as you increase the intensity of your activity the amount of fat that you use decreases
- as you increase the intensity of your activity the amount of glucose that you use increases
- there are numerous benefits to training and getting fit
- eating before you train decreases the amount of fat you burn
- training in the morning before you eat is an ideal way to burn fat

Exercise intensity

So far we have looked at almost everything there is to know about fat. We have discussed different types of fat, myths about fat, relationships between fat and a healthy life, and when the body uses fat as a source of energy. We will now look at the final piece to the fat jigsaw puzzle: *how fat is stripped during exercise*. Some fat-stripping activities have the potential to offload significant amounts of fat from the body's fat stores. The most important part of physical activity is firstly to do it at the correct fat-stripping intensity, and secondly to give yourself some time to assess your progress. There are plenty of theories about the best way to exercise for fat loss, but in the end there are only a few activities that actually work. There is a difference between exercising the heart, and hence keeping it healthy, and exercising so that your body strips fat from its storage sites. Exercise for fat stripping is not rigorous, painful or extremely intense. In fact it's quite the opposite.

Scientific evidence points to low-intensity activity as the best way to strip fat. The most effective fat-stripping activities are walking at a good pace and very light jogging. Cycling is also beneficial. Walking at a good pace means at a pace that causes you to puff after only a very short time – not a slow casual meander around the block, but a good, long-striding power walk. It is important to lift your heart rate in order to burn significant amounts of fat. If you wanted to jog, then this too should be done at a pace that allows you to maintain a good breathing rhythm even though you are puffing slightly.

You should be able to speak clearly while you jog. If you choose to cycle, then this also needs to be done so that you are puffing slightly, and just able to talk. The longer you do these activities the more fat you will strip. The graph below shows the relative amounts of fat and glucose used during different intensities of exercise. You can see that while sprinting uses the most energy, walking or other low-intensity exercise uses the most fat.

The body burns up roughly three times as much energy during strenuous exercise as it does during walking. High-intensity activities such as sprinting or weight lifting, which can be maintained for only ten to twenty seconds, use more energy (glucose) but much less fat. However, the body uses much more

PERCENTAGE OF FAT AND GLUCOSE USED AT DIFFERENT INTENSITIES

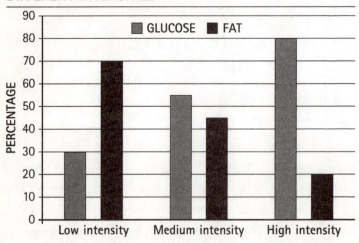

fat than glucose during low-intensity exercise such as walking. At this pace the human body is very efficient at stripping and burning fat. So although running burns more kilojoules, walking burns more fat. Low-intensity exercise can be maintained for *much longer periods* than sprinting or other flat-out exercise because the energy (glucose) stores are not depleted so quickly as during flat-out training. The aim is to find a pace that is somewhere between walking and running, such as power walking or light jogging. Remember, it is important to have variety in your exercise, so that it fits easily into your lifestyle. For example, walk one day, rollerblade the next, and then maybe cycle to a friend's house on the weekend.

One of the most important questions that needs to be asked before you choose an exercise is 'Will I burn fat while doing it?' There are some general rules you should follow to optimise your fat-burning activities. If you keep these in mind whenever you exercise, then you will have a clear understanding of when your body is burning fat.

1 If you are participating in an exercise and you become extremely short of breath, then you are using mainly glucose.

2 Remember that whenever there is an explosive burst of energy, the use of large amounts of fat is highly unlikely.

3 If you can do an activity continuously for a long period of time, and puff, but not too much, then you are most definitely using your fat stores.

Start off slowly

The question that you may ask is 'Why is fat used more at this low level?' Firstly, there is plenty of oxygen available for your body when exercising gently. This scenario is ideal for the body to use fat as a source of energy. In Chapter 4 we looked at the process of removing fat from the fat cells (lipolysis), and the burning of fat (oxidation). These vital functions can only happen when oxygen is present. The delivery of fat to exercising muscles takes some time, so you must be active for at least fifteen minutes before your body starts to use significant amounts of fat. The body cannot deliver fat as a fuel to the exercising muscles in an urgent rush. If your body needs a sudden burst of energy, if you were sprinting for the train, for example, then glucose is called into action. The mobilisation of glucose is much faster than that of fat. This means when exercising to strip fat from your fat stores you shouldn't be puffed out, but able to maintain a good breathing rhythm.

You can monitor that you are exercising at the optimal fat-stripping level by checking that you are not too puffed as you exercise. You shouldn't have any trouble getting your breath back when the activity is finished, and your legs shouldn't be heavy, as they would be after a fast sprint. If your legs feel too heavy during or after exercise, then you are moving too fast, and using glucose instead of fat.

At this low intensity, fat is continuously removed from its cells and supplied to the exercising muscles. As there is plenty of oxygen available, lipolysis and oxidation can function at optimal levels. As the graph (see page 88) shows, during low-intensity exercise the body can use fat to meet roughly 60–70 per cent of its energy needs. The remaining 30–40 per cent of energy is from glucose. An unfit person would initially use roughly 40–50 per cent fat as fuel, but with time this fat usage increases and could reach levels of 60–70 per cent. These are the main reasons why low-intensity exercise is highly recommended as being the most potent fat-stripping exercise.

Picking up the pace
Let's say that you were on your power walk and decided to pick up the pace. You are now into a good-paced run and are travelling at around 50–65 per cent of your fastest pace. This would be considered a moderate-intensity level. If you are a runner, then this pace is fine although you could not maintain this pace for a long period of time. If you are not a runner, then you may struggle to maintain a run at this intensity. This may in some ways be a positive, as the graph (see page 88) shows that when running at greater than half pace, the amount of fat used by the exercising muscles decreases. Although the body is using more energy when running at this higher pace, glucose, not fat, is the primary source of this energy. This is because the body cannot deliver fat fast enough to the exercising muscles in your legs. As you are breathing harder, there are decreased levels of oxygen, signifying a reduction in lipolysis. As there are lower levels of fat in the blood, there is obviously a decrease in the amount of fat delivered to the exercising muscles and hence less fat is burnt as

fuel. Glucose, on the other hand, can be delivered quickly and its use as a fuel is increased at this moderate intensity.

As the intensity of your exercise increases, more fast-twitch muscle fibres are used. Fast-twitch muscle fibres can provide a quicker release of energy than slow-twitch muscle fibres, which are predominantly used in lower-intensity exercises. In other words, fast-twitch muscle fibres are better equipped for burning carbohydrates than fat. As you move from a power walk into a run, the release of the hormone epinephrine is increased. This hormone helps in glucose breakdown and its use. Insulin is also present, so the level of fat in the blood decreases. This is an important point to take into account when choosing an exercise that helps you use fat. Jogging or fast walking lets the body burn more fat as fuel than moderate to fast running. Examples of moderate-intensity exercise may be a low- to high-impact aerobics class, cycling very fast on your bike, a short but semi-intense session on the step machine, or jogging up a hill. These exercises are, of course, good for overall fitness and cardiovascular health, but they are not the best or most effective way to remove fat from the body. Be aware also that jogging and running at a reasonable speed place a greater strain on the back and joints, and for the average person this can be dangerous. There are also the motivational factors associated in going for a fast run. It is not easy to set yourself a goal of running and pushing yourself. Studies have shown that this can actually be demotivational. It is much easier, and more beneficial for using fat, to walk at a good pace.

Absolutely flat out

Activities that require us to go flat out burn very little fat. During high-intensity exercise, the exercising muscles need energy in a mad rush and the body just cannot deliver fat fast enough to them. Fat is trapped inside its area of storage and cannot leave the fat cell. Hence during these activities even the first step of fat burning (lipolysis) is halted. The body can, however, deliver glucose to these muscles, so vast amounts of glucose, and not fat, are burnt as fuel. High-intensity activities include sprint training, cycling flat out during spinning classes, running extremely fast over a longer distance, weight training and boxing-type classes such as boxercise or tai bo.

Studies have also tested to see what would happen if free fatty acids were injected into the bloodstream during exercises of high intensity. Would the exercising muscle now use these fats that have been injected into the bloodstream? The answer is *not completely*. Only a small portion of these injected fats enter the muscle cells and are used as fuel. Something blocks the majority of fats from getting into the muscle cells to be burnt as fuel. High-intensity activity is clearly not conducive to burning fat. It seems that fat has trouble in getting to the furnace (the mitochondria), because carnitine's function is inhibited. Carnitine helps transport fats into the mitochondria where fat can be burnt as fuel. Carnitine is blocked by malonly-Co-A, an enzyme that increases its presence when glucose is in abundance. These are the basics of exercise metabolism.

As we now know, glucose levels can run out very quickly during exercise. This is why flat-out exercise can only be maintained for short periods of time. As with medium-intensity exercises, high-intensity activity is by no means bad for you. It is good for health and fitness, but if you are looking for immediate or long-term fat loss, then high-intensity training is not the way to go.

The myths of fat loss

There is always some new piece of equipment promoting fat loss launched on an already overloaded market. Some companies may claim that by doing a certain exercise you can actually burn more fat. You may have seen these companies advertising pieces of equipment or innovative training methods. Unfortunately, this just cannot be the case. People are fed up with purchasing equipment that they believe will burn more fat, and finding that it does no such thing. It is common to see these discarded fitness machines gathering dust as their promises are rarely fulfilled. In actual fact, no machine can make you burn more fat. These are indeed truly false claims and are a product of clever advertising.

As an individual, there are limits to how much fat you can burn, and this is determined by:

- the type of exercise you do
- the intensity at which you do it
- your genetics
- your fitness level

This of course doesn't mean that you cannot lose a lot of fat, but rather, losing body fat cannot be increased by a piece of fitness equipment. In this chapter we have discussed which exercises burn the most fat, and have shown that, contrary to popular belief, low-intensity activity of a long duration burns the most significant amount of fat. People think that they need to exercise hard and fast, and even punish themselves in order to burn fat and lose weight, but as demonstrated in this chapter, this is not the case. In understanding that fat loss can be achieved without 'strenuous' hard work, many people may be pleasantly surprised!

The only way to get rid of cellulite

Cellulite is fat, and the only way to get rid of cellulite is to work it off. This is stubborn fat that can be exercised off in the same way that fat is exercised off, with low-intensity exercise over a long period of time. There are many theories as to why cellulite seems to appear suddenly. Women always tell me that it came about 'all of a sudden'. One plausible explanation could be that while you are younger and more active, this activity, or a more active lifestyle, helps to use up more fat. Stopping or reducing physical activity can help bring about fat storage on the thighs and buttocks. I have found that a lot of women wait until they develop cellulite before they decide to start doing anything about it. Remember that cellulite is just fat and with plenty of walking, jogging or cycling you can reduce this fat and get rid of it once and for all.

Will sit-ups burn fat off my stomach?

'Spot reducing' is one of the greatest myths of physical exercise. For example, if you are doing sit-ups, which work your abdominal muscles, you are exercising the muscles but you are not necessarily reducing fat off your stomach. You lose fat only from the last place that you put it on. This means that while doing sit-ups you could actually be mobilising fat from your legs, arms or buttocks. By working your leg muscles you could even be utilising fat from your back. Sit-ups are by no means useless for reducing body fat, but they will not specifically reduce the fat on your stomach. It simply means that you need to continually exercise to mobilise all your body fat.

There is no special exercise or piece of equipment that will decrease the body fat in your abdominal region. *Everyone* has rippling abdominal muscles, and if you can't see them clearly it is because they are covered with abdominal fat. Exercise and a low-fat eating plan will help these muscles to become toned and the body to use up its excess fat.

The better you get

As you continue on your low-intensity training program you may find that the more you do, the less puffed you become. After some time you may find that the same walk that originally took you 45 minutes now takes you only 37 minutes, you are not so puffed and you don't sweat that much anymore either. You are getting fitter! Getting fitter in this way has many advantages. One of the greatest advantages with respect to the burning of fat is that as you become fitter, your body becomes better at using fat. If you are currently inactive, then you will burn less fat walking and running than shown in the graph on page 88. As you become more active, however, your body will start to use more fat and less glucose. In other words, your body develops a greater ability to take fat into the muscle cells, and to burn fat during exercise. This is a major adaptation the body makes to training. There are some major reasons for this adaptation:

- an increase in the number of enzymes responsible for fat burning
- an increased number and size of fat-burning sites (mitochondria)
- an increased use of fat that is already in the muscle
- an increased ability for muscle cells to take in fat to be burnt
- an increased ability for fat to be removed from its storage sites (adipose tissue)

As you become fitter and exercise more, your body can also increase its use of fat after exercise. This increased use of fat is needed during the recovery part of training, such as getting your body temperature back to normal, getting your breath back and restoring your glucose stores.

Should I eat before I train?

One of the most important considerations about training is asking yourself 'Do I want to lose fat?' What you eat before you train may affect how much fat or glucose you strip during exercise. Remember that during exercise you want to use fat as a fuel for your exercising muscles. The more fat you use, the less stays on your body!

Suppose, however, you eat a meal only one hour before you train. As you know, after a meal, the blood is abundant with glucose. This glucose needs to be pushed into the liver and muscle cells by insulin. When insulin is present, fat use dramatically decreases. Of course, if you now started to train, you would primarily use glucose and not fat. This is because you ate in the one-hour period before you trained, raising both the glucose and insulin levels in your blood.

Studies have shown that if you were to eat a piece of fruit or even a small bag of sweets before you were to embark on some fat-burning exercise, then the amount of fat that you would burn would decrease by 40–50 per cent. The significance of this for your eating and training means that your last meal or snack needs to be eaten roughly two hours before you train. This could mean that you eat a relatively large lunch at roughly 12.30 p.m., and then a snack at around 3.30 p.m., even if you are not hungry, and then exercise at around 6 p.m. Once again, to the elite athlete this may not mean too much, but to the average person trying hard to lose body fat then this is just another 5 per cent point that can help you. If you haven't eaten two hours prior to training, then have a sports drink or eat something straight after training. Drinking water at all times during your fat-stripping program is encouraged.

If we estimate a 40 per cent reduction in fat loss during exercise (due to eating two hours before training) and a 20 per cent increase in fat usage for recovery, then we can enhance fat loss significantly. The combination of healthy eating and increased training ensures that our bodies are meeting optimal conditions for fat stripping. If you are not taking these points into consideration, then you could decrease your fat usage by a conservative 35 per cent every day of its maximum potential. Over a period of weeks and months, this certainly adds up.

> Exercising before
> breakfast is a very
> effective way of
> fat stripping.

There is another alternative. Cyclists and runners who want to reduce their body fat levels exercise in the morning before they have eaten at all. Before breakfast is the best time to exercise and burn fat because studies show that insulin levels are low at that time. When insulin levels are low the body can use more fat as energy. A fast walk or light jog of roughly 40–50 minutes is an ideal scenario for fat loss. In fact if I could recommend a perfect time to exercise, then it would be in the morning. Apart from the enhanced fat stripping that can take place, it is a peaceful, noiseless time in which you can plan your day, concentrate, or even see the world when it is quiet. You will be also amazed at how hungry you become straight after training in the morning.

The effects of certain exercises on fat burning

There are many sports that people think are extremely beneficial for fat loss. Any form of exercise is great for general fitness and a healthy lifestyle, but as we have discussed, fast walking and gentle jogging are the best exercise for actual fat loss. You can always supplement these fat-loss activities with other sports that you enjoy or sports that will add a little more muscle tone to your body, if that is what you want. The important point when choosing a sport is to determine your goals. Do you just want to be fit or do you want to get rid of that fat?

Swimming

One of the most common misconceptions about exercise and fat loss is that swimming is a good activity for burning fat. Unfortunately for all those people who have raced out to purchase a new swimsuit, this is just not the case. Scientists have always been puzzled by the fact that swimmers don't seem to have the same low levels of body fat as their fellow elite athletes, such as runners and cyclists. Sports science has found that although swimming, running and cycling use the same amount of energy, recent evidence suggests that swimming uses more glucose for energy, while land training such as running and cycling utilises more fat. Swimming is a fantastic exercise for working your heart and developing your cardiovascular fitness, but it does not serve as an optimal exercise to reduce your body fat levels.

This can be clearly illustrated using two different elite athletes. We will use a swimmer, Kieren Perkins, and a track and field athlete, Carl Lewis. Kieren Perkins would train for many hours in the pool each day, and like his fellow swimming athletes Kieren would have approximately 10–12 per cent body fat. If you were to watch the finals of swimming events it would be common to see the eight finalists not being absolutely 'shredded' to the bone. The term 'shredded' refers to extremely low levels of body fat. Carl Lewis, on the other hand, would undergo the vast majority of his training through jogging and sprinting. He would not spend the same amount of time training as his swimming counterpart. He would, however, have approximately 5–6 per cent body fat. This level of body fat would be the same for the majority of track athletes, runners and elite cyclists. In fact, if you were to watch the final of a sprint or 800-metre race, you would see that all the athletes are very vascular, extremely lean and very shredded. You would think that a person such as Kieren Perkins, who spends many hours swimming as part of his training, would have a very low level of body fat. This is not the case.

In elite swimming when an athlete is carrying higher levels of body fat than desired, the athlete is sent back to what swimmers call 'land training'. This consists of running and cycling. Once the swimmer has lost significant amounts of body fat through a series of running and cycling, then swim training is recommenced.

There are other reasons that swimming may not be a fat-burning activity. While swimming, a person's body weight is supported by the water. This means that a person doesn't have to work as hard to move their body. As the water provides a cooler environment to train in, compared to walking, running or cycling, the body doesn't need to spend as much energy after exercise to get the temperature back to normal.

So in the scheme of things, I have omitted swimming from the optional fat-loss program, even though exercising by swimming can burn some fat (although not as much as other activities). Swimming can, however, be a part of an active lifestyle that supplements fat-burning activities.

Aerobics

In an aerobics class there may be times when you are exercising extremely hard, and you run out of breath. If this is a continual pattern throughout the class then you are probably not using a significant amount of your fat stores. In this case, you are better off trying a class of a lower impact, or doing some fast walking first, to build up your fitness. Once you have done this you may be able to do your aerobics class without running out of breath. After some time in one aerobics class, however, you may find that you are not puffing enough! Once you have got your fitness levels up, you may like to try a higher-intensity class, but remember that if you are running out of breath, then you are not burning fat at a first-rate level.

Pump, spinning and other high-intensity classes

There is now a variety of pump, boxing, karate and spinning classes in many gyms. Pump classes are circuit-type classes with weights, and spinning classes require you to cycle at different intensities on a stationary bike. Once again, if you remember our rules for fat loss, then these classes fall into the category of high-intensity. If the pump class was done with a light weight that didn't allow you to lift the weight until your arms drop off, then it might serve as a moderate- to high-intensity exercise and still burn fat. This, however, would still not be as effective as our low- to moderate-intensity training, but it can be extremely beneficial after your fat-burning work.

Golf and tennis

Although golf and tennis are fun to play, they too fail to aid in the burning of fat. If we consider the energy expended during tennis is explosive, requiring continual surges of power, followed by a rest, then unfortunately the rest far outweighs the running and hitting. Golf too requires small periods of explosive power followed by longer periods of slow walking. If the golfer power-walked in between the strokes, then golf might aid in fat loss, but unfortunately this doesn't usually happen. Once again, both activities are superb for maintaining a healthy heart and highly recommended as part of any active lifestyle, but they do little to help the body burn significant amounts of fat.

Weights and resistance training

Although weight training does not burn significant amounts of fat when compared to walking, it can actually be a very beneficial exercise. We have previously discussed the importance of increasing one's metabolism (see pages 96–7). One way of doing this is to increase the amount of muscle you have on your body. Walking and other low-intensity exercise will do this, but weight training enhances muscle gain even more (although this is not essential). The secret to doing weight training is to include it in your program *after* you have completed some low-intensity activity. This way you have developed a double-edged sword to your training. You have not only walked for say 45 minutes, but you've done some resistance work after this that will help increase your muscle mass.

For the average person starting off on this program, gym work or weight training is not essential, but as you become fitter you may like to work on increasing your tone and muscle mass. If you are a regular gym junkie, then consider this major change in your program. Some programs start with a 20-minute warm-up on the bike or walking machine and then some weight work taking around 30–40 minutes. The warm-up is not used primarily for fat burning, but as a way to get your body warm and loose for the weighted exercises. Here the emphasis is on the weight training. Much better is the concept of 45–60 minutes doing some fat burning like walking, light jogging or cycling, followed by 15–20 minutes of weight work. This puts the emphasis on the fat usage rather than the weight training.

Exercising in the heat

Exercising in the heat has the potential to cause injury. Some people think that by running, walking or cycling for long periods in warm conditions, they will lose more fat by sweating more. This is just not the case. In fact, they would most probably use less fat and more glucose than if it were cooler. Exercising in the heat can potentially lead to dehydration and heat stroke, especially when fluids are not consumed, or consumed only in small doses.

I have often seen people wear layers of clothing, including plastic garbage bags underneath their track suits, in the belief that they will shed more fat this way, as they will sweat more. Yes, they do sweat more, and if they weigh themselves before and after the run, the scales may show some weight loss, but this is just loss of water. As soon as you drink gallons of fluids (because you are dehydrated), the scales will show that you have regained the weight. On warm days, exercise in the cool of the morning or night.

Metabolism

Exercising will help you lose fat. If you follow this chapter carefully, then you have a sure-fire recipe for fat loss. Exercising will also increase your muscle mass. This is important, as if you have more muscle, then your body has to work harder to feed it, clean it, supply it with nutrients such as minerals and vitamins, and keep it in good condition. Your body expends more energy to carry out these functions, so the added muscle does actually speed up your metabolism. There are other ways in which your metabolism can be sped up. We will examine this in the next chapter (see page 109).

The key points to remember from this chapter are intensity and duration. Keep your exercise at a low-intensity level, and keep this pace going for as long as you can. If you are going to do high-intensity exercise, then do it after your low-intensity work.

SUMMARY:

- the best exercises for fat loss are low-intensity
- if you are puffing hard when exercising, you are not working at an ideal fat-stripping level
- any exercise is good for you, but to burn fat brisk walks are best
- exercise helps to improve your metabolism so that you burn fat faster

THE
FAT-STRIPPING
DIET

Key messages for this chapter

YOU WILL DISCOVER:
- that the success of your diet depends upon your preparation and planning
- that preparation includes menu planning and having plenty of recommended snacks handy
- that greater amounts of food can be eaten when they are low in fat
- that alternative food choices can be made for breakfast, lunch and dinner
- hints for eating out
- recommended snack foods

Putting it all together

This is the chapter that puts everything that we've looked at so far into a practical and workable perspective. There is something very exciting and exhilarating about starting a new diet or embarking on a new challenge. Hopefully this will be your first step into a healthy and profitable lifestyle change. What's even more exciting is checking the date on your calendar, and finding that you've been cruising along on your diet for a month and are not missing anything about your previous eating habits. Wouldn't it be fantastic to find that the diet that you started on is no longer a diet but rather 'just the way you eat now'. The Fat-Stripping Diet is not a seasonal diet, you can use it all year round. Ideally, you will adopt this program as a healthy, permanent way of life. This is a diet that can be used effectively by almost anyone, and one that *will* decrease your body fat. Much of the information in this chapter relates to the seven-day eating plan at the end of the book (see pages 154–9). The principles of the diet are discussed here, so you know exactly what you are eating and why, then once you set out on your fat-burning program you can be guided by the eating plan.

If you have read all the chapters so far, then you yourself are somewhat of an expert on fat loss. You now know all that there is to know about fat, and how the body responds when you eat it. You also know the physical cost of eating fat. The physical cost of fat really puts fat into perspective as never before. You should also have a fundamental understanding of the best way to exercise to burn important fat energy. These are the answers to the questions that I had years ago. You now have just about all these answers. With all this in mind it is now up to you to make some important decisions. You will have several choices to make.

This diet must be one of the few that actually gives you the option of eating chocolate and sweets. As this diet is designed for you to lose fat, it doesn't mean that you will be hungry or starve or have an eating plan based on prunes and carrots. There are no special foods that you need to eat, and there are no special foods that you continually need to buy. Foods do not need to be eaten in special combinations or ratios, and there are no New Age mystical hormones that we are going to tap into via this diet. This diet is a successful one, and my clients have been very happy, because the results have been long-term ones. This diet also allows you to boost your metabolism by providing smaller portions of food at more regular intervals throughout the day.

The aim of this chapter is to provide you with plenty of low-fat food options, to keep you from reaching your fat surplus. We have previously discussed how the body needs only a certain amount of fat to function. Any amount of fat greater than this required amount will be stored as body fat. By following the sample diet provided here you will fall well within your 41 grams or 60 grams of necessary fat each day. If you follow this diet correctly, then your body will be searching for fat to use as fuel. In doing so it will turn to your fat stores and your body's fat levels will start to dwindle. If you have eaten extremely well all day and your fat intake is only 11 grams, you could, if desired, eat a small chocolate bar. Your fat intake would be 20 grams for the day, but if you were to do this every so often it would not hinder your fat-loss goals.

The principles of the Fat-Stripping Diet

The Fat-Stripping Diet is one that aims to reduce fat by cutting down on fatty foods in your diet. The Fat-Stripping Diet is based on a maximum fat intake of just 15–20 per cent. This means that 15–20 per cent of the body's energy comes from fat that you eat during the day. The rest of the energy should come from carbohydrates and stored body fat.

On the Fat-Stripping Diet:

- Protein is *not* used as an energy source.
- Carbohydrates such as fresh fruit and vegetables, whole-grain breads, cereals, rice and pasta will *not* be converted to fat.
- In the amounts that have been recommended, these foods will be converted into glucose and then into glycogen. This glycogen will then be stored in your liver and muscle cells.
- You will not be overeating on carbohydrates.
- This is not a super-high-carbohydrate, super-low-protein diet, but rather a diet that balances the energy needs and the growth needs of the body.
- The body will spend large amounts of energy breaking down carbohydrates, transporting and storing them.

- As carbohydrate will be used for energy, protein will be used for its specific functions (see page 31).
- As your body has enough energy from the daily intake, you will not lose valuable muscle mass. Remember that the more muscle you have on your body, the more sites there are for fat to be burnt.
- You will have plenty of energy and won't feel lethargic.

All my clients follow the Fat-Stripping Diet, with excellent results. The diet has been shown to be incredibly effective over a ten-week period. Naturally, those clients who have maintained the diet for a longer period of time have had even better results with fat stripping. In ten weeks, most clients lose at least 5 kilograms, the bulk of which is fat, while others lose considerably more when they have really kept their fat intake to an absolute minimum.

The difference with this diet is that once the fat weight is off it stays off. Unlike other diets where, as soon as you finish dieting, the weight comes rushing back on, the Fat-Stripping Diet promises permanent fat loss. This diet removes body fat and not good-quality muscle, which is usually the first thing to go in crash diets. When clients have followed the eating plan (see pages 154–9) and then decided to become active, or more active, it is not uncommon to see more dramatic weight loss, roughly 10–12 kilograms over a ten to twelve week-period. The most positive aspect of this diet is that it is so easy to fit it into any lifestyle, and it soon becomes second nature.

Determining the minimum of fat that the body needs has been at the forefront of modern nutritional physiology, and numerous studies that allow us to measure fat metabolism have been completed. It is important to understand that when we talk about the minimum amount of fat that the body needs, we are talking about an estimated value. This value will be different for every individual, so it is important that we use this value only as an estimated guide. It is not necessary to reduce the fat intake to lower than 15–20 per cent as the body requires some fat in the diet, especially in the form of essential fatty acids, to function optimally. For the majority of people, fat sources are topped up every day because they eat so much fat. This means that the body will store this excess fat unless it is exercised off.

Let's examine three very different diets. One diet was very high in fat (60 per cent of the energy came from fat), one diet was high in fat but similar to the way we eat in Australia (40 per cent of energy from fat), and the third diet was the one that we are following in this book (roughly 20 per cent of energy from fat). The results of this study can be seen in the table below.

GRAMS OF FAT CONSUMED PER DAY

PERCENTAGE OF FAT IN DIET	FEMALE	MALE
20	41 grams	60 grams
40	82 grams	120 grams
60	123 grams	180 grams

(Adapted from Stubbs, Harbron, and Prentice, 1995)

FAT LOSS OR GAIN PER WEEK

	20% FAT IN DIET	40% FAT IN DIET	60% FAT IN DIET
Week 1	125	75	450
Week 2	250	150	900
Week 3	500	225	1350
Week 4	750	300	1800
Week 5	1100	375	2250
Week 6	1400	450	2700
Week 7	1700	525	3150
Week 8	2200	600	3600
TOTAL	2200 grams lost	600 grams gained	3600 grams gained

The body uses fat as a source of energy, so if the fat intake is reduced, then the body will draw this energy from stored body fat. Without doing any physical activity, those people who were on the 20 per cent fat diet spontaneously lost real body fat. After only one day on this diet, the people involved actually lost 50 grams of body fat. This would be difficult to measure, and you might not even notice that it was gone, but if you were to use the Bilsborough Fat Cost Chart, you would see that women need to walk for 160 minutes or 17 kilometres to work off that amount of fat. Men need to walk for 119 minutes or 12 kilometres to work of 50 grams of fat. After four days the subjects had lost over 125 grams of fat, which equates to about half a kilogram of weight loss per week. This may not seem much but it translates to healthy, permanent weight loss. Not only would the '20 per cent fat eaters' be losing fat weight, but also a fair amount of body weight. In eight weeks their bodies' metabolisms would have used up over 2 kilograms of fat, which translates to roughly 6–8 kilograms of body weight. This is why it is important to be patient with your diet.

If we look at the figures for the people who were on the 40 per cent fat diet, we see a gradual rise in the amount of fat stored. It is interesting to note that these people had stored no body fat after 3 days. In one week, the body had gained a total of 75 grams of fat. This may not seem like much, and in the scheme of things it isn't. This is just one bad week, but over a longer period of time the amount of surplus fat would be quite large. As with the people who were on the 20 per cent fat diet, these subjects didn't know that they had put on weight after just one week. After eight weeks the situation for the '40 per cent fat eaters' isn't so bad – their fat storage is estimated to be 600 grams. In weeks ahead, however, this would have accumulated even further.

> It is important
> to be patient
> with your diet.

The people on the high-fat diet put on 100 grams of fat in only two days. An addition of 100 grams of body fat would hardly be noticeable, and this is how we actually put on fat. Little by little, week by week, this small amount adds up. In only a short space of time kilograms of fat are put on and this is where it becomes noticeable. In seven days this rose to over 450 grams. In four weeks this has amounted to nearly 2 kilograms. Interestingly, this group considered themselves to be eating normally, and not eating a diet high in fat. This may be a case where people have trouble identifying how much fat is in food. It is important to have a rough understanding of the fat values of food, as the most frustrating thing would be to be actually eating more fat than you planned. Once again it must be remembered that people on all three types of fat intakes didn't exercise and all thought that they were eating normally.

The eating plans

I love food and I love to eat. The most important thing about this diet is that you should really enjoy the food and meals that you are eating. No-one is going to stick to a diet if the food is awful or bland, so the Fat-Stripping Diet provides a wide of variety of menus and food choices. And it is flexible.

The format of the diet is based on smaller meals at more regular intervals. This means eating six meals during the day, which is lighter than the conventional three big meals. It is important to keep eating throughout the day. This is called grazing. Graze only on the foods that have been recommended. The eating plans (see pages 154–9) show the maximum amounts that I recommend you eat. Some people will find that there is too much food on the menu, so if you cannot eat all the recommended food for the day, eat what you can without overdoing it. Once again, these amounts are the limits.

For the female tables, there is enough calcium and iron in these eating plans to meet the recommended daily intakes. Red meat should be eaten two to three times per week to meet iron needs, with plenty of low-fat milk, low-fat yoghurt and low-fat ice cream incorporated for calcium requirements. The diet allows you to stay within your 41 grams and 60 grams of fat per day, if you follow it carefully. In fact the total fat for the women following the diet is 147 grams in six days. This is an average of 24.5 grams per day. If you are trying to stay just under 41 grams per day you can do so with ease. You are roughly 16.5 grams under this mark every day. If a male were to follow this diet, he would have eaten 143 grams of fat in six days. This averages out to roughly 24 grams of fat per day. This is a remarkable 36 grams of fat below our mark of 60 grams per day. Following this diet for six days, the average male would have eaten only 143 grams of fat in total. If he had eaten exactly 60 grams per day he would have amassed 360 grams per week. This is nearly 220 grams below our target per week.

With this in mind, read the list of foods provided on pages 154–9 carefully, and when you are next in the supermarket buy a week's worth of groceries. Preparation is the key to your success. Always be prepared for your next day's eating.

Alternatives: you know the cost, now make the choice
When you are conscious of what you are eating, one of the pitfalls is eating the same food all the time and getting bored. Eating plans need to have a large variety of food that you can choose

from. Below are some alternatives for every meal, so you can have an interesting and varied diet. If you do eat the same thing all the time, chances are you will lash out and binge on a hamburger and chips or chocolate biscuits. You now know the shockingly high-fat costs of certain foods. You need to be aware of these mammoth fat costs when you are choosing items to eat. Have plenty of choices handy to stave off becoming bored with a diet!

Breakfast kick-starts your metabolism in the morning and provides you with essential energy to start the day. Don't miss it!

BREAKFAST OPTIONS

- low-fat cereal
- untoasted muesli
- oats or porridge
- toast with jam, marmalade, honey or vegemite and a very light scraping of margarine, or better still no butter or margarine at all
- low-fat muffins with jam
- muffins with cottage cheese or honey
- poached eggs on toast
- toasted ham and tomato sandwich
- two bananas and yoghurt
- banana smoothie (using two bananas and low-fat milk)
- glass of Sustagen (if you don't feel like eating in the mornings)

Making and packing your lunch before you go to work is the key to sticking to this diet. Poor preparation will lead to poor eating habits and won't help you lose any fat. All these meals form the basis of your lunch, and remember that there are always one or two pieces of fruit and a drink you can have with your meal. Some people may find that they are unable to eat all the food recommended for each meal. If you find that one sandwich is too much then don't force yourself to eat a whole one.

LUNCH OPTIONS

- bowl of soup with 3–4 pieces of bread
- bruschetta, plenty of fresh tomatoes, basil and no cheese or oil
- toasted sandwiches (no cheese and no spreads or fillings that have been preserved in oil)
- sandwiches, especially with turkey filling, are very low in fat (only 4 grams)
- pita bread with salad or ham or chicken filling
- chicken or tuna salad with 2–3 pieces of bread
- homemade caesar salad using lean bacon and low-fat caesar salad dressing (no cheese). Have some bread with this meal
- medium bowl of reheated low-fat pasta from the night before with some salad
- any reheated leftovers that are low in fat
- baked beans on toast is a very healthy meal. If you use very light scrapings of margarine on the toast then this meal will also be low in fat
- steak sandwiches are good for a weekend lunch. Grill thin slices of steak and fry some onions in very small amounts of oil. Top with tomato, lettuce and maybe an egg (no cheese)

As with all other aspects of this diet, remember that planning is the key. You may come home tired and not inclined to stick to your good eating plan, but if you are prepared, then eating a low-fat evening meal is easy.

DINNER OPTIONS

- lasagna (use lean mince)
- chicken or vegetarian pasta
- steak sandwich
- roast lamb or beef with vegetables (including potatoes)
- Vietnamese rice paper rolls
- large bowl of vegetable soup with bread (4–5 pieces)
- chicken and vegetable stir-fries with rice
- beef or lamb stir-fries or curries (with vegetables) served with a large bowl of rice. Use this as an alternative to steak and vegetables. Serve larger amounts of rice and vegetables with smaller amounts of meat

Like all of us, I really dislike going hungry. Grazing during the day is good, but snack on the right stuff. If you find at any time that you are going hungry (which you shouldn't), choose something filling from the healthy snack suggestions. Keep plenty of snacks around the house or in your drawer at work. Of course, these snacks should not be seen as a substitute for the pieces of fruit included in the eating plans, but if every now and then you want a change or still feel a little hungry, then you are allowed something different. As you become more accustomed to this diet and become better at reading food labels, you will be able to add other low-fat but tasty snacks to your list.

SNACKS

- bread and jam
- muesli bars (low-fat)
- fruit sticks
- jelly babies or snakes
- Milky Way chocolate bars (only 4.3 grams of fat)
- Turkish Delight (1 every two days)
- low-fat sweet biscuits
- low-fat scones
- rice puddings (low-fat)
- rice crackers with low-fat cottage cheese
- rice crackers with salsa
- baked beans
- milk shakes (low-fat)
- banana smoothies
- frozen yogurt
- low-fat yogurt

Eating out

Most people can manage eating at home and work reasonably well. When we dine out, however, this becomes very difficult. Most of the time we are left to guess whether the plate of sweet and sour pork and fried rice is really doing us good. How bad is it? Most of the time when people are watching what they eat they feel guilty on birthdays, or special occasions, or with friends going out to a restaurant. They feel that this has wrecked the diet that they have been following religiously for the last month. Don't ever feel embarrassed to ask how the chef is preparing your meal or to request a low-fat option. On many occasions I have asked for steamed vegetables rather than stir-fried or roast vegetables with my meal, even if they don't appear on the menu. This is how you can control your fat intake.

If you have a business lunch, then you can swap your lunch for dinner. Have a piece of grilled steak or grilled fish with steamed vegetables. You can turn this situation into a positive, as you then don't have to cook a big meal at night. You can then just have a sandwich and some soup with bread rolls for dinner.

The Fat-Stripping Diet gives you a night off each week.

One night off the diet each week allows you to have flexibility in your lifestyle and will encourage you to stick to your diet. Don't feel guilty if you are dining out while on the fat-stripping diet. This is actually encouraged. While dining out, however, there are certain ways in which you can minimise your fat intake.

If you have followed the diet closely then you will have eaten much less than the recommended 41 or 60 grams of fat per day. This will mean that for women, potentially, at the end of the week, you could be 140 grams under the mark of 287 grams (7 × 41). Men could be 252 grams under the mark of 420 grams (7 × 60). In this case, after you have been following the eating plan for five to six weeks, you could afford a night out on the town worth 60–80 fat grams! Of course, you might not want to totally undo all the good work of the week, but the aim here is to find a balance between following the diet and living a 'normal' lifestyle.

Weekends

In the eating plan for Saturday, sushi or nori rolls have been suggested for dinner (see page 159). It is assumed that you are dining out for this meal, in which case choose any kind of low-fat option. Sushi is ideal. If you are eating at home, choose a meal from any of the dinner options. Sunday is also left free, to give you more flexibility. You may have a long lunch with friends and just a small salad for dinner. See how you feel; you may like to follow a particular day's eating plan or you might choose to mix and match from the breakfast, lunch and dinner options (see pages 117–19). Hopefully you will do this with the understanding of the energy costs of these foods. The idea again is to allow you greater flexibility between your diet and your lifestyle.

Alcohol

Alcohol consumption yields only 'empty calories' because it provides no essential vitamins or minerals to the body.

Although alcohol can be consumed while on the fat-stripping diet, it must be consumed only in moderation. The term moderation does not mean two to three glasses of wine a night and a whole bottle on Saturday night. Moderation means one glass per night. If you reduce the amount you drink you will be better off in terms of fat loss. There is some suggestion that when consumed in moderation, some alcohol such as red wine may be helpful in reducing cardiovascular disease, so don't feel guilty about your diet for drinking a glass of wine with dinner.

All other processes of the body, including fat stripping, are put on hold while alcohol is broken down and released. This breakdown of alcohol happens at a slow rate as only a certain amount can be broken down at any one time. This is why when you drink too much it takes a long time to 'sober up'. Alcohol is absorbed into the blood and rushed to the liver. Roughly 80 per cent of alcohol, or ethanol, is converted to a substance called acetate and sent to muscle cells where it can be burnt as fuel. This process takes the place of fat oxidation and hence less fat is burnt for energy. While alcohol is being metabolised the release of fat into the bloodstream is inhibited. Fats are not released from their fat cells, and hence the fat-burning process is reduced.

Alcohol can contribute to your energy needs during the day, but there are several disadvantages. The main problem with drinking alcohol during any diet is that it has a high energy content, and most of the time alcohol is served alongside fatty junk food such as chips and nuts. These foods are only snacks, but if you look at their energy costs you will find that these items take a lot of time to burn off. Once again, moderation (one standard drink per day) is the key.

SUMMARY

- the Fat-Stripping Diet is based on 15–20 per cent of the body's energy requirements coming from fat
- the foods you eat should be varied and interesting
- the Fat-Stripping Diet is flexible
- you shouldn't go hungry if you follow the eating plans (see pages 154–9)
- use the snacks only as a last resort
- you have one night off each week from the Fat-Stripping Diet
- by following the diet, you will lose weight safely and permanently

FAT FREE –
A LEANER BODY

Key messages for this chapter

YOU WILL DISCOVER:

- that supplementing your diet with some exercise can strip even more fat from your fat stores
- that having one bad day is not a disaster if you have eaten and exercised well during the rest of the week.
- exactly how much fat you can burn through diet and exercise together
- that the best and most effective way to strip fat is to walk fast
- that using the Bilsborough Fat Cost Chart (see pages 162–5) can help you work out how much fat you would burn during any amount of walking

Getting back to fat balance

In Chapter 7 we examined what happened to a group of people who had three types of diets (see pages 112–15). One diet was very high in fat and consisted of 60 per cent of energy from fat. The second diet derived 40 per cent of its energy from fat, which was still considered to be a diet high in fat. The third diet was one that derived 20 per cent of energy from fat. This last diet is almost identical to the fat-stripping diet, which has a total fat intake of 15–20 per cent. This diet allowed for the 20 per cent fat to be used by the body. The body then looked for other fat to use as energy and started eating away at the stored fat. It was found that these people then lost body fat. This fat loss was described as 'spontaneous' and 'gradual'. The diet that consisted of 40 per cent fat resulted in slight fat accumulation, and the 60 per cent, high-fat diet resulted in rapid fat gain. These results were measured when these people were totally inactive.

It is startling to realise
just how much of an
impact exercise has
on fat loss.

If you wanted to boost your diet even further, and help your body use even more fat, then you need to be more active. This does not mean that you have to join a gym, take up aerobics or become a fitness freak. Being active means that you may start walking briskly two or three times a week if you were doing no exercise at all before. When the people on the low-fat (20 per cent) diet started exercising, the amount of fat removed from their bodies was quite significant over a fourteen-day period. It is startling to realise just how much of an impact exercise has on fat loss. This was true even for the subjects who had a diet that consisted of 40 per cent fat. In fourteen days these subjects were also well under their fat balance when they were active. The people who followed a diet that was very high in fat still had stored fat after they began exercising, but the amount of fat stored in fourteen days while being active was less than half as much of the fat that was stored after seven days of no exercise at all. All these groups of people lost two to three times as much fat once they started to exercise. In two weeks, the people on the 20 per cent fat intake diet had lost 725 grams of fat. The people on the 40 per cent fat intake diet had lost 220 grams.

The amount of exercise you do is totally up to you, but by the time you've finished this chapter, you may be thinking that walking several times per week is a very good idea. The tables in this chapter show how exercising can greatly influence the amount of fat lost each day for men and women. The Bilsborough Fat Cost Chart (see pages 162–5) shows how much fat men and women use during these exercise times. Of course, these values will vary from person to person, but they give you an indication of the relationship between exercise and fat loss. Being able to actually observe how eating and exercising affects how much fat we use up is a very useful and motivational tool.

Fat loss in men and women

Let's see how different lengths of exercise can improve the amount of fat the body uses for the day. The female body needs a maximum amount of fat of 41 grams each day. If Sarah eats 15 grams of fat then the body still needs 26 grams (41 – 15) for the day for energy, which it finds by eating away at her fat stores (column 2). The total amount of fat used for the day (column 6) is found by adding how much fat her body needs (column 2) to how much fat her body uses during exercise (column 5). We can see from this table that the longer you exercise, the more fat your body uses. The amounts of fat used during exercise are found using the Bilsborough Fat Cost Chart (see pages 162–5).

WOMEN

FAT EATEN (grams)	FAT BALANCE (grams) 41 – (column 1)	EXERCISE	TIME (minutes)	FAT USED (grams)	TOTAL BODY FAT USED FOR DAY (grams) (column 2) + (column 5)
15	41–15=26	walking	30	5	26+5=31
15	41–15=26	walking	45	9	26+9=35
15	41–15=26	walking	60	15	26+15=41

The table clearly shows that if Sarah were to do even a little exercise, she would already increase the amount of fat that her body uses for the day. The more exercise of low-intensity and long duration, the more fat she uses. As column 6 shows, good-pace walking can make fat loss even more significant. Sarah would have begun to lose body fat in her first week of the Fat-Stripping Diet but probably doesn't know it. If you've been walking or cycling or more active in general, then as long as you have followed the eating plan you will have definitely lost fat!

Men need a maximum of 60 grams of fat in their diet each day. If you are following the eating plans, your fat intake will be much less than this, and your body will turn to stored fat to provide the extra energy required. By adding exercise to this program, you are significantly influencing your fat loss.

MEN

FAT EATEN (grams)	FAT BALANCE (grams) 60 – (column 1)	EXERCISE	TIME (minutes)	FAT USED (grams)	TOTAL BODY FAT USED FOR DAY (grams) (column 2) + (column 5)
20	60–20=40	walking	30	7	40+7=47
25	60–25=35	walking	45	15	35+15=50
40	60–40=20	walking	60	20	20+20=40

The Fat-Stripping Diet takes into account that people are busy at work and at play, and have different energy levels at different times. You may have a really good week where you walk every morning or every night, followed by a week where you just don't get a chance to exercise. You may have some good days and some bad days. You may even think that the total fat lost or stored in each table is not significant enough to persist with the eating and exercise program. This is why people give up walking, light jogging or cycling, and take up more strenuous exercise. They feel that they need to push themselves harder. They want dramatic weight loss immediately but the faster you go, or the more intensely, the less fat you burn. This is a *fat-stripping* diet. Use the tables in this chapter as a guide for your own exercise routine together with the eating plans, and you will be pleased with your toned, fat-free body.

Exercise plans for women

In a good week such as presented in the table below, Sarah manages to walk four times and eat well every day. Two mornings she walked her dog, and twice she walked with a friend. Sarah burnt an extra 48 grams of fat by including exercise

A GOOD WEEK

DAY	FAT EATEN (grams)	FAT BALANCE	EXERCISE	TIME (minutes)	FAT USED (grams)	TOTAL BODY FAT (grams)
MON	15	41–15=26	walking	60	15	41 lost
TUE	22	41–22=19	none			19 lost
WED	21	41–21=20	walking	45	9	29 lost
THU	22	41–22=19	none			19 lost
FRI	25	41–25=16	walking	45	9	25 lost
SAT	22	41–22=19	none			19 lost
SUN	24	41–24=17	walking	60	15	32 lost
TOTAL	151	136		210	48	184 lost

in her program. She has done two important things: she has stuck to her diet and supplemented her diet with some exercise. Maybe 184 grams in a week doesn't seem like much but it is important to remember that this is fat loss. This is very different from muscle loss, water loss and weight loss. Fat loss of 184 grams every week for three months is 3–4 kilograms, which translates to about 10–12 kilograms in permanent weight loss.

AN EVEN BETTER WEEK

DAY	FAT EATEN (grams)	FAT BALANCE	EXERCISE	TIME (minutes)	FAT USED (grams)	TOTAL BODY FAT (grams)
MON	15	41–15=26	walking	60	15	41 lost
TUE	22	41–22=19	walking	60	15	34 lost
WED	21	41–21=20	walking	60	15	35 lost
THU	22	41–22=19	none			19 lost
FRI	25	41–25=16	walking	60	15	31 lost
SAT	22	41–22=19	none			19 lost
SUN	24	41–24=17	walking	60	15	32 lost
TOTAL	151	136		300	75	211 lost

In this particular week (above) Sarah has managed to walk five times. In total she has used up roughly 211 grams of fat from her body as energy. This value of 211 grams may not seem significant, and may not even be noticed, but if this kind of lifestyle were to be maintained for several weeks or even months, Sarah would undoubtedly be a lot leaner.

Sarah didn't exercise this week, but from Monday to Thursday she still ate very well; therefore her body used approximately 84 grams of fat. Her weekend was not so good as she ate out on Friday and Saturday and went out for lunch on Sunday. Sarah didn't bother to follow the Fat-Stripping Diet's eating out options so she consumed a large amount of fat. For many of us this may be a typical weekend. Sarah has stored fat this week, but only 69 grams. She probably doesn't even notice that she has put on this fat, even though she would be feeling guilty about breaking her diet.

EATING WELL BUT NO EXERCISE

DAY	FAT EATEN (grams)	FAT BALANCE	EXERCISE	TIME (minutes)	FAT USED (grams)	TOTAL BODY FAT (grams)
MON	15	41–15=26	none			26 lost
TUE	22	41–22=19	none			19 lost
WED	21	41–21=20	none			20 lost
THU	22	41–22=19	none			19 lost
FRI	117	41–117=–76	none			76 stored
SAT	60	41–60=–19	none			19 stored
SUN	99	41–99=–58	none			58 stored
TOTAL	356	69				69 stored

Remember that one bad week is just not as bad as you think. We may feel guilty because we have eaten the wrong food, but the damage in terms of the bigger picture may not be so bad.

Exercise plans for men

Simon tried but couldn't stay under his allocated 60 grams of fat per day this week. In everyday terms, he has still done a fantastic job as this was one of his busy weeks – he still managed to prepare his lunch, and he exercised three times during this week. During a week such as this Simon is still able to lose some body fat. As the table shows, any man who really wants to make a fist of fighting fat can! One of my clients went from 107 kilograms to 85 kilograms over a fourteen-month period through sheer determination.

AN AVERAGE WEEK

DAY	FAT EATEN (grams)	FAT BALANCE	EXERCISE	TIME (minutes)	FAT USED (grams)	TOTAL BODY FAT (grams)
MON	60	60–60=0	walking	60	20	20 lost
TUE	60	60–60=0	none			0
WED	60	60–60=0	walking	60	20	20 lost
THU	60	60–60=0	none			0
FRI	60	60–60=0	walking	60	20	20 lost
SAT	60	60–60=0	none			0
SUN	60	60–60=0	none			0
TOTAL	420	0		180	60	60 lost

Supposing Simon ate quite a high-fat diet, close to his 60 grams of fat every day, and still exercised three times during the week. If this were maintained for three to six months, then the amount of fat and weight lost would be roughly 7–10 kilograms. Don't be harsh on yourself if some weeks aren't as good as others. These not-so-good weeks can be rather good weeks when you see how much fat is still being lost.

At the end of this week of eating well and exercising three times, Simon has lost just over 300 grams. He may not notice this fat loss, but nevertheless it is substantial, and one week of good eating is a fantastic foundation to build on. I'm sure many people have been eating correctly but, because they couldn't assess their fat loss, simply gave up. These tables show that if it is fat loss you want, then start tomorrow. Once again, using the Bilsborough Fat Cost Chart (see pages 162–5), we can determine how much fat Simon would use during a walking time of 60 minutes.

EATING WELL AND EXERCISING

DAY	FAT EATEN (grams)	FAT BALANCE	EXERCISE	TIME (minutes)	FAT USED (grams)	TOTAL BODY FAT (grams)
MON	23	60–23=37	walking	60	20	57 lost
TUE	31	60–31=29	none			29 lost
WED	24	60–24=36	walking	60	20	56 lost
THU	23	60–23=37	none			37 lost
FRI	24	60–24=36	walking	60	20	56 lost
SAT	22	60–22=38	none			38 lost
SUN	25	60–25=35	none			35 lost
TOTAL	172	248		180	60	308 lost

In an excellent week of eating and exercising, Simon, like almost any other male, can reduce his level of body fat. As the table below shows, this can amount to almost 350 grams per week, and if this were to be maintained for several months then Simon would have indeed decreased his body fat levels, as well as his total body weight. As these scenarios have clearly demonstrated, even during weeks where you cannot exercise, if you follow the diet plan, then you will still lose real body fat.

AN EXCELLENT WEEK

DAY	FAT EATEN (grams)	FAT BALANCE	EXERCISE	TIME (minutes)	FAT USED (grams)	TOTAL BODY FAT (grams)
MON	23	60–23=37	walking	60	20	57 lost
TUE	31	60–31=29	walking	60	20	49 lost
WED	24	60–24=36	walking	60	20	56 lost
THU	23	60–23=37	walking	60	20	57 lost
FRI	24	60–24=36	walking	60	20	56 lost
SAT	22	60–22=38	none			38 lost
SUN	25	60–25=35	none			35 lost
TOTAL	172	248		300	100	348 lost

A bad week

When Sarah and Simon eat badly, by keeping up a high-fat diet, they store this fat each week. Even though they exercise, the vast abundance of fat they are consuming during these weeks is too much to work off, and far in excess of what their bodies can use. As we have continually stressed, this is just one of those weeks. A new day will dawn tomorrow, and with it a shift away from eating too much fat.

What if I exercise well, but eat badly?

The average Australian woman eats about 70–80 grams of fat per day (1995 National Dietary Survey). The average Australian male eats roughly 120 grams of fat each day. If Sarah and Simon, like a lot of people, think that exercising three times per week gives a licence to eat anything they want, they should think again. Even if a person exercised all week but ate a diet that had an average of 70 or 120 grams of fat per day, they would store fat.

What if I have a bad weekend, but exercise a lot?

Exercise is the only thing that can offset the negative effects of what you've eaten. If you are headed towards a big weekend, and decide that you are not going to be able to stick to your diet, then you may need to exercise for five days during the week. The remarkable thing is that if Sarah walked during all five days, then she would still have lost fat during the course of the week. This seems like hard and unnecessary work. You are better off watching what you eat on the weekend, but of course sometimes these situations cannot be avoided. A typical example of this is if you are going to a party and you guess that there may not be very healthy food available. Christmas and office parties can sometimes be unavoidable and so, in keeping with the theme of the Fat-Stripping Diet – be prepared! How many of us simply throw a whole week away because we had a bad weekend or a few bad days? If you know you won't be able to eat well, you can make a concerted effort to increase the amount of activity you do during the week. Rather than giving up and letting the whole week be a bad one, you can also decide to stick to the eating plan specified by the Fat-Stripping Diet.

Being active

Being active doesn't always mean that you have to be an athlete, or go jogging every second day. There are many other ways that your body can spend energy. Being active basically means you need to keep moving. If you are stuck behind a desk all day or lounging in front of the television, then you're probably not helping your situation in terms of spending energy.

The best and most effective way to exercise

Without a doubt the most effective way to lose fat is by fast walking. If you can jog or ride a bicycle, then a combination of three exercises can be beneficial. As we have already discussed, keep the intensity low to moderate. The more you can do the better; however, this requires some motivation. There is a method that may help you solve this problem. It's called *cycling*. It has nothing to do with a bicycle and is an extremely effective way of staying fit and motivated.

Athletes cycle their training by having times when they train maybe five times a week, and times when they may only train twice a week. Following this type of structure, your exercise cycle may look like the following:

EXERCISE PYRAMID

week 1	walk 2 times
week 2	walk 3 times
week 3	walk 3 times
week 4	walk 4 times
week 5	walk 3 times
week 6	walk 3 times
week 7	walk 2 times
week 8	rest

This is called a pyramid cycle: one that builds up the amount of times you train each week and then reaches a peak, in this case week 4. Once at this peak the amount of times you exercise decreases. In an eight-week cycle you can have a week off. This cycle can be written as a 2, 3, 3, 4, 3, 3, 2 pyramid.

You could try others that are more intense and stay at the peak for a lot longer. A pyramid of this sort might be a 2, 3, 4, 4, 4, 5, 5, 4, 4, 4, 3, 2 pyramid. It is important to have some structure to your exercise plan. Just exercising on a whim is not effective planning, and does nothing to complement your fantastic diet. Setting small weekly and monthly goals can also help you get a firm grip on where you are with fat loss. For example, you can make it a point to record the amount of time and distance and fat grams that you burn up each week. Make it your goal to increase these values every week.

SUMMARY
- exercising will greatly influence fat loss
- don't give up after one bad day
- plan your exercise for the week ahead
- weight loss *can* be achieved without exercise, but exercise can further enhance fat loss
- although you may not notice much fat loss after one week, persistence over a ten-week period will lead to a well-toned, leaner body
- in the long-term, you will have the body shape you want

STAYING MOTIVATED

Motivation

Finding the motivation to stay on track can be very difficult. Sometimes situations arise that are totally out of your control, such as an unexpected dinner invitation, or going to a party that serves junk food for the entire evening. It's situations like these that can make us feel that sticking to the diet just isn't working, or worth it. With the Fat-Stripping Diet this is surely not the case. One bad day isn't the end of the world; neither is one bad week. In the last chapter we saw the consequences of a bad week, and in the grand scheme of things it is really no big deal. Sometimes having a bad day is good motivation to do the right thing for the next few days or weeks. The bottom line is that you need to keep pushing forward. The foods on the meal plan are probably no different from what you have been eating during the week anyway, apart from a few minor adjustments here or there, and of course a new and clearer understanding of fat.

Getting started is the hardest part, but this can also be an exciting time. If you start this diet with a friend or group of friends then it will be easier for you in the long term. Find a consistent walking or exercising partner who will motivate you to exercise, even when you just don't feel like it. Having worked as a fitness advisor and personal trainer (amongst other things) for many years, I have found the main reason for being hired was for motivation. In fact, one of my longest-standing clients (of nearly six years) says that his motivation to get up and train is that I am at his doorstep at six o'clock in the morning. If he wasn't paying me to be there, he says he just wouldn't get up. Initially this was difficult but now it is just a part of his life. Having a personal trainer is a great idea, if you are really struggling for some motivation. If you feel that personal trainers are too expensive, get a group together, and that way the rates are cheaper. Other ideas are to get your own group of friends together, even just two or three, and each morning get up and out and catch up while walking together.

Other sources of motivation should come from what you learnt in Chapter 6. That chapter let you know how much damage you are doing to yourself in terms of fat storage, not to mention the effect on cholesterol, blood pressure and heart disease. Almost everyone I speak to is concerned with what foods are doing to him or her. People have not been able to understand exactly what eating even small amounts of fat can do. Chapter 6 of this book should shock you and hopefully motivate you to make some real household changes. Some of the distances that need to be walked in order to lose certain amounts of fat are quite daunting. Rather than walk those distances, stay away from these high-fat foods. By this stage you should have a good grasp of the way fat is stored and burnt as fuel. This should also be a source of motivation to keep you going on the right track.

> Time is the key.
> The longer you stay
> on this diet, the more
> fat you will lose.

Planning

On numerous occasions throughout this book I have used the word 'preparation'. This is the key to successful fat loss and weight reduction. If you are not prepared with your meal planning, then you are planning to fail. When you consider that planning your meals for the week takes around ten minutes, and making your lunch takes about eight minutes, it really isn't so difficult. Some clients with whom I have worked closely have found that writing out something as simple as a shopping list has been helpful. Another helpful hint is never to go shopping when you are hungry. It is too easy to buy food that isn't on the menu guide and you would probably also buy too much.

Spending some time in a supermarket, studying the nutritional labels on food packets, may also help you find delicious low-fat alternatives. Before leaving home in the morning make sure that you have enough food for mid-morning, lunch and mid-afternoon. Plan to have food – snack food, good food and more good food – at home, at work and in your handbag or briefcase, as well as in your car if you drive.

Assessment

If you have been following the diet correctly then you will undoubtedly be losing body fat. Numerical assessment in this case may be difficult unless you have access to a pair of skinfold calipers. These calipers can be used to monitor the change in fat and muscle on your body. The ultimate in fat reduction, however, will appear on the scales in the long term. My own father came to me asking how he could reduce his enormous belly. Without having any other form of measurements, he would ring me up each month telling me that his pants were too big around the waist, and how he needed to cut new holes in his belts. This is without doubt the best form of measuring the success of your diet. My father was so scared of exercising the long distances that were described in Chapter 6 that he thought he would just stick to the diet. In six months he had lost 15 kilograms, and now (twelve months later) he has stabilised with a total loss of 17 kilograms.

Although my father is only one example, you may lose weight at a different rate, either faster or slower. Rapid weight loss is not recommended, as most of the time the weight lost is in the form of muscle. Fat loss is more gradual, and can be a more permanent form of weight loss. Remember that somewhere in your journey there may come a sticking point or plateau phase. It may be that your body has stabilised or adapted to or become used to what you are doing. It means that you need to change things around more. For example, you may need to walk faster as you are getting fitter. You could change things around by cycling for two weeks, and then cycle and walk. You could walk, jog lightly and then cycle just to add some variety to your program. If you are only dieting and not exercising, there will come a time when you are no longer burning large amounts of fat. At that point you will need to boost your program by exercise. Remember how much more fat the subjects in Chapter 7 used when they started being active!

Time and patience

I once worked as both a fitness advisor and nutritionist for a corporate executive. A lifestyle management consultant may have been a better term for the job. When we first started our lifestyle plan he weighed 110 kilograms with a body fat of around 32 per cent. In the first couple of weeks he said he didn't feel that he had lost any fat, and sometimes his body-weight went above 110 kilograms. This is typical of many people, who think that after exercising for a little while they feel they haven't lost anything. In actual fact, my client's body fat had reduced to 29 per cent when I measured it even though his bodyweight was still 110 kilograms after about a month.

What had happened was that although he actually lost 3 per cent body fat (over 3 kilograms of fat) by walking, he had increased his muscle mass from 75 kilograms to 78 kilograms. In the following period of fifteen months he went on to be 90 kilograms with 17.5 per cent body fat. All we did in this time was walk. The point is that because things don't seem to be working, it doesn't mean that they are not. Give yourself time and I tell you sincerely that you will not be disappointed.

> Time is the golden
> ingredient that really
> makes your diet and
> exercise work for you.

The sad thing is that so many people give up in just two or three months because they think there have been only small changes. On many occasions when I measure body fat levels during the course of an exercise and diet program that I have set, these people are amazed at the change in their fat and muscle mass. Once they know this, then all of a sudden they are on a high and can recognise the small changes.

This book boils down to taking responsibility for the way you eat and the way you look. The Fat-Stripping Diet is certainly not a fad, and combined with regular, low-intensity exercise, it will ensure an even leaner, more toned body. Your diet is where fat accumulation begins. If you understand that fat is the real danger in our eating and not sugar or complex carbohydrates, then you are well on the way to success.

APPENDICES

Key to tables in this chapter:

- energy costs of common and high-fat foods
- energy costs of fast foods
- the Fat-Stripping Diet 7-day eating plan
- self-use chart
- the Bilsborough Fat Cost Chart for men and women

ENERGY COST OF SOME COMMON AND HIGH-FAT FOODS

Here are some foods that are most commonly consumed in the Australian diet. Here, also, are some of the foods we feel most guilty about eating. Not surprisingly, many of these foods are very high in fat and take a mammoth amount of time to work off your body. Remember that if your fat intake is less than 41 or 60 grams per day – as it is with the Fat-Stripping Diet – then you don't need to worry about the minimal amount of fat that is contained in bread or rice; these small amounts are burnt up by the body's metabolism and are factored into your fat allowance of 41 or 60 grams.

The following tables show the fat values, and their implication, of only the most basic foods. If you are serious about fat stripping, it is a good idea to invest in a comprehensive fat counter, available from any bookshop. Then, when you are planning your meals, you can use the Bilsborough Fat Cost Chart (see pages 162–165) to work out how far you need to walk and how much time this would take to work off any fat and to keep your body lean.

FOOD	FAT (grams)	WOMEN		MEN	
		WALKING TIME (minutes)	WALKING DISTANCE (kilometres)	WALKING TIME (minutes)	WALKING DISTANCE (kilometres)
▶ DAIRY butter (1 tablespoon)	15	59	6.2	48	4.4

continued

FOOD	FAT (grams)	WOMEN		MEN	
		WALKING TIME (minutes)	WALKING DISTANCE (kilometres)	WALKING TIME (minutes)	WALKING DISTANCE (kilometres)
▶ DAIRY – *continued*					
margarine (1 tablespoon)	15	59	6.2	48	4.4
full-cream milk (1 glass)	10	45	4.7	36	3.5
low-fat milk (1 glass)	0	0	0	0	0
soy-milk (1 glass)	9	41	4.3	34	3.2
thickened cream (1 tablespoon)	7	36	3.8	30	2.7
plain yoghurt (1 small tub)	8	40	4.2	33	3
cheddar cheese (1 cube)	5	30	3.2	25	2.3
scrambled eggs	15	59	6.2	48	4.4
▶ GRAINS & CEREALS					
white bread (1 slice)	1	18	1.7	15	1.4
brown bread (1 slice)	1	18	1.7	15	1.4
multi-grain bread (1 slice)	1	18	1.7	15	1.4
pasta (100 g)	1	18	1.7	15	1.4
rice (100 g)	0	0	0	0	0
muffin	11	48	5	38	3.7
muesli bar (full-fat)	4	27	3	23	2.1
croissant	15	59	6.2	48	4.4
▶ MEAT & FISH					
2 lamb chops, grilled, fat on	30	103	10.9	83	7.5
2 lamb chops, grilled, fat trimmed	11	48	5	38	3.7

continued

FOOD	FAT (grams)	WOMEN		MEN	
		WALKING TIME (minutes)	WALKING DISTANCE (kilometres)	WALKING TIME (minutes)	WALKING DISTANCE (kilometres)
▶ MEAT & FISH – *cont*					
1 small beef steak, grilled, fat on	26	90	9.4	74	6.5
beef, fat on (¾ cup, diced)	19	70	7.3	58	5.4
beef, fat trimmed (¾ cup, diced)	12	50	5.2	41	3.8
2 sausages, grilled	23	83	8.9	66	5.8
veal schnitzel, fried	39	130	13.6	110	9.9
½ chicken breast, skin on, baked	12	50	5.2	41	3.8
2 bacon rashers, grilled, fat on	13	52	5.5	44	4.1
fish, crumbed and fried	10	45	4.7	36	3.5
tuna, canned in oil (1 cup)	28	96	10	80	7.2
tuna, canned in brine (1 cup)	5	30	3.2	25	2.3
▶ SNACK FOODS & CONDIMENTS					
peanuts, salted (¼ cup)	21	78	8	62	5.6
potato crisps, (1 packet)	16	62	6.4	50	4.6
peanut butter (1 tablespoon)	13	52	5.5	44	4.1

continued

FOOD	FAT (grams)	WOMEN		MEN	
		WALKING TIME (minutes)	WALKING DISTANCE (kilometres)	WALKING TIME (minutes)	WALKING DISTANCE (kilometres)
▶ SNACK FOODS & CONDIMENTS – *cont*					
mayonnaise (1 tablespoon)	7	36	3.8	30	2.7
doughnut, iced	19	70	7.3	58	5.4
rich cream sponge (1 slice)	15	59	6.2	48	4.4
chocolate biscuit	5	30	3.2	25	2.3
Wagon Wheel	8	40	4.2	33	3
chocolate block (6 squares)	8	40	4.2	33	3
jelly babies	0	0	0	0	0
▶ FRUIT & VEG.					
avocado (¼)	14	55	5.9	46	4.2
apple	0	0	0	0	0
banana	0	0	0	0	0
carrot	0	0	0	0	0
potato	0	0	0	0	0
▶ DRINKS					
fruit juice	0	0	0	0	0
lemonade	0	0	0	0	0
red wine	0	0	0	0	0

ENERGY COST OF FAST FOODS

FOOD	FAT (grams)	WOMEN		MEN	
		WALKING TIME (minutes)	WALKING DISTANCE (kilometres)	WALKING TIME (minutes)	WALKING DISTANCE (kilometres)
Big Mac	24	86	8.9	70	6.2
Cheese Burger	13	52	5.5	44	4.1
Quarter Pounder with Cheese	26	90	9.3	74	6.5
Whopper	39	130	13.6	110	9.9
Bacon Double Cheese Burger	39	130	13.6	110	9.9
Bacon and Egg McMuffin	19	70	7.3	58	5.4
McDonald's Big Breakfast	31	105	11.5	85	7.5
Zinger Burger	17	65	7.2	52	4.8
Chicken Fillet Burger	22	75	8.6	60	5.9
Chocolate Sundae	9	41	4.3	34	3.2
Caramel Sundae	8	40	4.2	33	3
Thick Shake, large	13	52	5.5	44	4.1
Lean Cuisine beef goulash	10	45	4.7	36	3.5
Lean Cuisine chicken carbonara	11	48	5	38	3.7
Lean Cuisine satay lamb	12	50	5.2	41	3.8
Lean Cuisine Thai chicken curry	12	50	5.2	41	3.8
Maggi 2 minute noodles, 1 packet	16	62	6.4	50	4.6
satay beef	25	88	9.1	72	6.1
chicken basil	27	95	9.9	75	7.1
chicken curry	18	69	7.1	55	5

continued

FOOD	FAT (grams)	WOMEN		MEN	
		WALKING TIME (minutes)	WALKING DISTANCE (kilometres)	WALKING TIME (minutes)	WALKING DISTANCE (kilometres)
beef in oyster sauce	20	75	7.7	60	5.4
fried noodles	19	70	7.3	58	5.4
fried rice	15	59	6.2	48	4.4
garlic prawns	14	55	5.9	46	4.2
hot chilli beef	22	81	8.6	64	5.9
lemon chicken	22	81	8.6	64	5.9
moussaka	20	75	7.7	60	5.4
taco	21	78	8	62	5.6
pizza (1 slice)	13	52	5.5	44	4.1
pizza with extra cheese (1 slice)	16	62	6.4	50	4.6
quiche (1 slice)	25	88	9.1	72	6.1
cannelloni	22	81	8.6	64	5.9
lasagna	14	55	5.9	46	4.2
dim sim, deep-fried	5	30	3.2	25	2.3
plain hamburger in bun	17	65	6.9	52	4.8
1 meat pie	26	90	9.4	74	6.5
Four'n Twenty pie	21	78	8	62	5.6
party pie	4	27	3	23	2.1
sausage roll	23	83	8.9	66	5.8
sausage roll (party size)	8	40	4.2	33	3
potato chips, hot	13	52	5.5	44	4.1

THE FAT-STRIPPING DIET 7-DAY EATING PLAN

Remember that this diet is very easy to follow. There are no extremes – you don't starve, you don't overload on carbohydrates and you don't cut out protein altogether. The Fat-Stripping Diet is designed to give you enough energy to get you through the day, while still reducing your fat intake so that enough fat can be stripped to give you a lean body. It keeps your fat intake well below 41 grams for women and 60 grams for men. The seven-day eating plan contains foods that will meet all your fibre, vitamin, mineral, essential fatty acid and protein requirements. In particular, this diet provides the necessary daily intake of calcium (800–1200 mg) and iron (10–20 mg) for women.

The diet consists of approximately 55–60 per cent carbohydrates which, according to the Bilsborough Fat Cost Chart (see pages 162–165), takes no time to walk off as it is not fat! Many of these carbohydrates are in the forms of healthy, nutritious foods, such pasta, rice, bread, cereals, potatoes, fresh fruits and vegetables. After three to four weeks of following this eating plan you can look at the Breakfast, Lunch and Dinner options (see pages 117–19) and incorporate these meal suggestions into your diet. As you become more confident with how you manage your eating, you will be able to introduce a huge variety of interesting, tasty and low-fat foods into your diet.

MON ▶	WOMEN	MON	MEN
mealtime	food	mealtime	food
breakfast	2 Weet-Bix with low-fat milk (250 ml) 1 orange	breakfast	3–4 Weet-Bix with low-fat milk (250 ml) 1 orange
snack	1 banana 1 low-fat muesli bar	snack	1 banana 1 low-fat muesli bar
lunch	1 ham and salad roll (no cheese) 1 apple	lunch	1–2 ham and salad rolls (no cheese) 1 apple
snack	1 tub low-fat yoghurt 1 fruit juice (250 ml)	snack	1 tub low-fat yoghurt 1 fruit juice (250 ml)
dinner	1 fillet snapper, steamed pumpkin mashed potato broccoli 1 glass red wine (optional)	dinner	1 fillet snapper, steamed pumpkin mashed potato broccoli 1 glass red wine (optional)
dessert	1 small bowl frozen yoghurt	dessert	1 medium bowl frozen yoghurt

TUE ▶	WOMEN	TUE	MEN
mealtime	food	mealtime	food
breakfast	1 bowl of rolled oats with low-fat milk (250 ml) 1 orange	breakfast	1 large bowl of rolled oats with low-fat milk (250 ml) 1 orange

Appendices

mealtime	food
snack	3–4 water crackers with low-fat cottage cheese
lunch	1 tuna or salmon and salad roll (no cheese) 1 apple 1 diet soft drink
snack	1 low-fat muesli bar 1 banana
dinner	1 piece lean steak, grilled mashed potato carrots boiled spinach
dessert	2 scoops low-fat ice cream

mealtime	food
snack	3–4 water crackers 1 banana
lunch	1–2 tuna or salmon and salad rolls (no cheese) 1 apple 1 diet soft drink
snack	1 fruit juice (250 ml) 1 low-fat muesli bar 1 banana
dinner	1 piece lean steak, grilled mashed potato carrots boiled spinach
dessert	2 scoops low-fat ice cream

WED	WOMEN
mealtime	food
breakfast	2 pieces toast with scraping of margarine and strawberry jam low-fat milk (250 ml)
snack	1 apple ¼ cantaloupe
lunch	1 tuna or salmon and salad roll (no cheese) 1 diet soft drink

WED	MEN
mealtime	food
breakfast	2 pieces toast with scraping of margarine and strawberry jam low-fat milk (250 ml)
snack	1 apple ¼ cantaloupe
lunch	1–2 tuna or salmon and salad rolls (no cheese) 1 diet soft drink

mealtime	food		mealtime	food
snack	1 orange		snack	1 banana 1 orange
dinner	1 small bowl pasta with low-fat tomato-based sauce and tuna or salmon		dinner	1 medium/large bowl pasta with low-fat tomato-based sauce and tuna or salmon
dessert	1 bowl fruit salad		dessert	1 bowl fruit salad

► THUR	WOMEN		THUR	MEN
mealtime	**food**		**mealtime**	**food**
breakfast	2 Weet-Bix with low-fat milk (250 ml)		breakfast	3–4 Weet-Bix with low-fat milk (250 ml)
snack	1 tub low-fat yoghurt with strawberries		snack	1 tub low-fat yoghurt with strawberries
lunch	1 ham and salad roll (no cheese) 1 diet cola		lunch	1–2 ham and salad rolls (no cheese) 1 diet cola 1 low-fat muesli bar
snack	1 banana 1 orange		snack	1 banana 1 orange
dinner	1 small bowl pasta with low-fat tomato-based sauce and extra lean mince green salad (with lots of spinach)		dinner	1 medium/large bowl pasta with low-fat tomato-based sauce and extra lean mince green salad (with lots of spinach)
dessert	1 bowl low-fat vanilla custard		dessert	1 bowl low-fat vanilla custard

Appendices

FRI	WOMEN	FRI	MEN
mealtime	food	mealtime	food
breakfast	1 bowl low-fat cereal or muesli with low-fat milk (250 mls)	breakfast	1 bowl low-fat cereal or muesli with low-fat milk (250 mls)
snack	1 banana 1 low-fat muesli bar	snack	1 banana 1 low-fat muesli bar
lunch	1 ham and salad roll 1 fruit juice (250 ml) 1 orange	lunch	1–2 ham and salad rolls 1 fruit juice (250 ml) 1 orange
snack	3–4 water crackers with low-fat cottage cheese or serving of salmon/tuna/or yoghurt	snack	3–4 water crackers with low-fat cottage cheese or serving of salmon/tuna/or yoghurt
dinner	1 piece lean steak, grilled mashed potato carrots spinach, boiled	dinner	1 piece lean steak, grilled mashed potato carrots spinach, boiled
dessert	2 scoops low-fat ice cream	dessert	2 scoops low-fat ice cream

SAT	WOMEN	SAT	MEN
mealtime	food	mealtime	food
breakfast	2 bananas mixed with 1 tub low-fat yoghurt	breakfast	2 bananas mixed with 1 tub low-fat yoghurt
snack	1 low-fat muesli bar	snack	1 low-fat muesli bar

mealtime	food
lunch	1 ham and salad roll
snack	optional: choose from list of snacks (see page 120)
dinner	sushi with seafood or 4–6 nori rolls with tuna 2 glasses red wine (optional)
dessert	1 Turkish Delight chocolate

mealtime	food
lunch	1–2 ham and salad roll
snack	optional: choose from list of snacks (see page 120)
dinner	sushi with seafood or 6–8 nori rolls with tuna 2 glasses red wine (optional)
dessert	1 Turkish Delight chocolate

Self-use chart

Setting up your own chart is very easy. If you have been following the Fat-Stripping Diet correctly then you will undoubtedly be under the fat surplus value of 41 grams for women and 60 grams for men. Assume the values of between 20 and 33 for women and 40 for men as the amount of fat you have eaten for the day. Place these values on your chart in column 2. The next thing to do is to take these values away from 41 or 60. Put these numbers in column 3. Write down the exercise and next to it the amount of time. Use the Bilsborough Fat Cost Chart (see pages 162–5) to estimate the amount of fat you burnt up during this exercise. Put this value in the column labelled 6. Now add column 3 and 6 for each day. You can also add up the time, fat burnt during exercise and total fat lost for the week. Try to improve these values each week. Photocopy this chart before you begin each new week on the Fat-Stripping Diet.

WOMEN: ONE WEEK OF FAT-STRIPPING

	FAT EATEN (grams) (2)	FAT BALANCE 41 – [2] (3)	EXERCISE	TIME (minutes)	FAT USED (6)	TOTAL BODY FAT USED (grams) = (3)+(6)
MON						
TUE						
WED						
THU						
FRI						
SAT						
SUN						
TOTALS						

MEN: ONE WEEK OF FAT-STRIPPING

	FAT EATEN (grams) (2)	FAT BALANCE 60 – [2] (3)	EXERCISE	TIME (minutes)	FAT USED (6)	TOTAL BODY FAT USED (grams) = (3)+(6)
MON						
TUE						
WED						
THU						
FRI						
SAT						
SUN						
TOTALS						

Using the Fat Cost Chart

Using the Bilsborough Fat Cost Chart on the following pages is quite simple. Most of us read the nutritional labels on food packaging to check the amount of fat in each product before we purchase it. Knowing that each gram of fat will correspond to a walking distance and time, you can use the graph to determine roughly how far and for how long you need to walk, given any amount of fat. You can also use this chart to note how much exercise you don't have to do!

When using the chart you will need to add up the total fat grams, the total times and distances for each individual food. Each food has a walking time and distance calculated for it, and each calculation takes into account a 15–20-minute time factor (the time it takes for the body to start using significant amounts of fat). This is the correct way to total up the energy cost of food. Obviously, you don't need to walk for the entire amount of time specified or cover the calculated distance; these graphs simply help you to understand just how much work you need to do to work off your fat intake. It is recommended that you reduce your fat intake in the first instance and then you won't store it.

By reading off how long and how far it takes to burn off individual foods, it can give you a rough idea of the cost of the food. To find out how much exercise you should do to avoid storing fat, add up your total fat intake for the day, subtract 41 or 60 grams from the total, then calculate your walking distance and time using the chart. This chart can also be used in reverse. For example, if you go for a fast walk for 50 minutes and want to know roughly how much fat you burnt then you simply go to the time axis and read off the corresponding amount of fat. Remember these values may differ for each individual and provide a rough guide rather than an exact figure.

How to read the fat cost chart:
1. Go to the amount of fat in a food, for example 15 grams.
2. From this value move up in a straight line until you touch the diagonal.
3. Draw a line across to read the values on the two vertical axes.
4. If the fat consumed is 15 grams, then a man needs to walk for 52 minutes or cover 5 kilometres. For the same amount of fat, a woman needs to walk for 60 minutes or cover 6.8 kilometres.

With this simple method, you can also work out how much fat you will lose if you walk for 45 minutes, for example, or cover 4 kilometres.

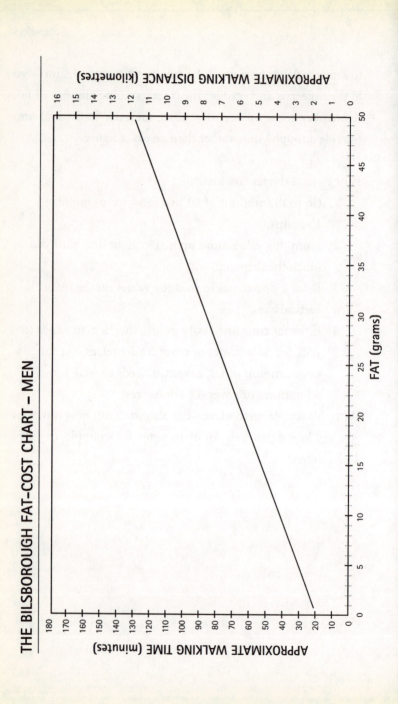

THE BILSBOROUGH FAT-COST CHART – MEN

APPROXIMATE WALKING DISTANCE (kilometres)

APPROXIMATE WALKING TIME (minutes)

FAT (grams)

THE BILSBOROUGH FAT-COST CHART – WOMEN

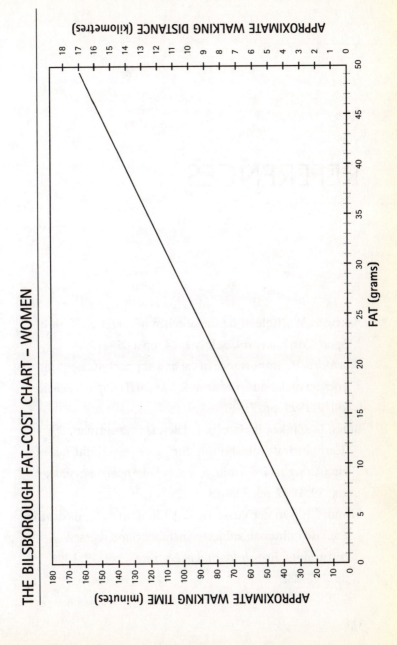

APPROXIMATE WALKING DISTANCE (kilometres)

APPROXIMATE WALKING TIME (minutes)

FAT (grams)

REFERENCES

Askew, E. W., 'Role of fat metabolism in exercise', *Clinic of Sports Medicine*, vol. 3, July 1984, pp. 605–21.

Bjorntorp, P., 'Importance of fat as a support nutrient for energy: metabolism of athletes', *Journal of Sports Science*, vol. 9, 1999, pp. 71–6.

Bracy, D., Zinker, B., Jacobs, J., Lacy, D., Wasserman, D., 'Carbohydrate metabolism during exercise: influence of circulating fat availability', *Journal of Applied Physiology*, vol .79, 1995, pp. 506–13.

Brounss, F., van der Vusse, G. J., 'Utilisation of lipids during exercise in human subjects: metabolic and dietary constraints', *British Journal of Nutrition*, vol. 79, 1998, pp. 117–28.

Brown, M. S., Goldstein, J. L., 'How LDL receptors influence cholesterol and atherosclerosis', *Scientific America*, vol. 251, 1984, pp. 52–60.

Cameron-Smith, D., Egger, G., Stanton, R., 'The effectiveness of popular, non-prescription weight-loss supplements', *Medical Journal of Australia*, vol. 171, 1999, pp. 604–8.

Charlton, M., Adey, D., Sreekumaran Nair, K., 'Evidence for a catabolic role of glucagon during an amino acid load', *Journal of Clinical Investigation*, vol. 98, No. 1, July 1996, pp. 90–99.

Cortright, R. N., Dohm, G. I., 'Mechanisms by which insulin and muscle contraction stimulate glucose transport', *Canadian Journal of Applied Physiology*, vol. 22, 1997, pp. 519–30.

Coyle, E. F., 'Substrate utilisation during exercise in active people', *American Journal of Clinical Nutrition*, vol. 61, 1995, pp. 968S–979S.

Coyle, E. F., Jeukendrup, A.E., Wagenmakers, A. J., Saris, W.H., 'Fatty acid oxidation is directly regulated by carbohydrate metabolism during exercise', *American Journal of Physiology*, vol. 273, 1997, pp. E268–E275.

Doucet, E., Tremblay, A., 'Food intake, energy balance and body weight control', *European Journal of Clinical Nutrition*, vol. 51, 1997, pp. 846–55.

Giugliano, D., Marfella, R., Verrazzo, G., Acampora, R., Coppola, L., Cozzolino, D., D'Onofrio, F., 'The vascular effects of L-arginine in humans', *Journal of Clinical Investigation*, vol. 99, No. 3, February 1997, pp. 433–438.

Hargreaves, M., 'Interactions between muscle, glycogen and blood-borne glucose during exercise', *Exercise Sports Science Review*, vol. 25, 1997, pp. 21–39.

Hargreaves, M., Kiens, B., Richter, E. A., 'Effect of increased plasma fatty acid concentrations on muscle metabolism in exercising men', *Journal of Applied Physiology*, vol. 70, 1991, pp. 194–201.

Hargreaves, M., McConnell, G., Proietto, J, 'Influence of muscle glycogen on glycogenolysis and glucose uptake in humans' *Journal of Applied Physiology*, vol. 78, 1995, pp. 288–292.

Hayashi, T., Wojtaszewski, J. F., Goodyear, L. J.,' Exercise regulation of glucose transport in skeletal muscle', *American Journal of Physiology*, vol. 273, 1997, pp. E1039–E1051.

Hellerstein, M. K., 'De novo lipogenesis in humans: metabolic and regulatory aspects', *European Journal of Clinical Nutrition*, vol. 53, Suppl. 1, 1999, pp. S53–S65.

Hepel, P., Vergauwen, L., Vandenberghe, K., Richter, E. A.,' Significance of insulin for glucose metabolism in skeletal muscle during contractions', *Diabetes*, vol. 45, 1996, pp. S99–S104.

Holt, S., Miller, J., Petocz, P., 'An insulin index of foods: the insulin demand generated by 1000-kj portions of common foods', *American Journal of Clinical Nutrition*, vol. 66, 1997, pp. 1264–76.

Horowitz, J., Mora-Rodriguez, R., Byerley, L., Coyle, E.,

'Lipolytic suppression following carbohydrate ingestion limits fat oxidation during exercise', *American Journal of Physiology*, vol. 273, 1997, pp. E768–E775.

Hutber, C. A., Rasmussen, B. B., Winder, W. W., 'Endurance training attenuates the decrease in skeletal muscle malonly-CoA with exercise', *Journal of Applied Physiology*, vol. 83, 1997, pp. 1917–1922.

Jequier, E., 'Response to and range of acceptable fat intakes in adults', *European Journal of Clinical Nutrition*, vol. 53, Suppl. 1, 1999, pp. S84–S93.

Jeukendrup, A. E., Saris, W. H., Schrauwen, P., Brouns, F., Wagenmakers, A. J., 'Metabolic availability of medium – chain triglycerides coingested with carbohydrates during prolonged exercise', *Journal of Applied Physiology*, vol. 79, 1995, pp. 756–762.

Kiens, B., Kristianson, S., Jensen, P., Richter, E. A., Turcotte, L. P., 'Membrane associated fatty acid binding protein (FABPpm) in human skeletal muscle is increased in endurance training', *Biochemistry and Biophysics*, vol. 231, 1997, pp. 463–465.

Linn, T., Santosa, B., Gronemeyer, D., Aygen, S., Scholz, N., Busch, M., Bretzel, R. 'Effect of long-term dietary protein intake on glucose metabolism in humans', *Diabetologia*, vol. 43, 2000, pp. 1257–1265

Martin, W. H., 'Effects of acute and chronic exercise on fat metabolism', *Exercise Sports Science Review*, vol. 24, 1996, pp. 203–31.

Maughan, R. J., Greenhaff, P. L., Leiper, J. B., Ball, D., Lambert, C. P., Gleeson, M., 'Diet composition and the performance of high-intensity exercise', *Journal of Sports Science*, vol. 15, 1997, pp. 265–275.

Miller, S. L., Wolfe, R. R., 'Physical exercise as a modulator of adaptation to low and high carbohydrate and low and high fat intakes', *European Journal of Clinical Nutrition*, vol. 53, Suppl. 1, 1999, pp. S112–S119.

Murray, R., Bartoli, W. P., Eddy, D. E., Horn, M. K., 'Physiological and performance responses to nicotinic-acid ingestion during exercise', *Medicine and Science in Sports Exercise*, vol. 27, 1995, pp. 1057–1062.

Patti, M., Brambilla, E., Luzi, L., Landaker, E., Kahn, C., 'Bidirectional modulation of insulin action by amino acids', *Journal of Clinical Investigation*, vol. 101, No. 7, April 1998, pp. 1519–1529.

Phillips, S. M., Green, H. J., Tarnopolsky, M. A., Heigenhauser, G. F., Hill, R. E., Grant, S. M., 'Effects of training duration on substrate turnover and oxidation during exercise', *Journal of Applied Physiology*, vol. 81, 1996, pp. 2182–2191.

Prentice, A. M., Poppitt, S. D., 'Importance of energy density and macronutrients in the regulation of energy intake', *International Journal of Obesity*, Suppl., 1996, pp. S18–23.

Romijn, J. A., Coyle, E. F., Sidossis, L. S., Zhang, X. J., Wolfe, R. R., 'Relationship between fatty acid delivery and fatty acid oxidation during strenuous exercise', *Journal of*

Applied Physiology, vol. 79, 1995, pp. 1939–1945.

Saha, A. K., Vavvas, D., Kurowski, T. G., Apazidis, A., Witters, L. A., Shafrir, E., Ruderman, N. B., 'Malonyl-CoA regulation in skeletal muscle: its link to cell citrate and the glucose fatty acid cycle', *American Journal of Physiology*, vol. 272, 1997, pp. E641–E648.

Sidossis, L. S., Gastaldelli, A., Klein, S., Wolfe, R. R., 'Regulation of plasma fatty acid oxidation during low and high-intensity exercise', *American Journal of Physiology*, vol. 272, 1997, pp. E1065–E1070.

Spiller, G.A., Jensen, C.D., Pattison, T.S., Chuck, C.S., Whittam, J.H., Scala, J., 'Effect of protein dose on serum glucose and insulin response to sugars', *American Journal of Clinical Nutrition*, vol. 46, 1987, pp. 474–80.

Spriet, L. L., Maclean, D. A., Dyck, D. J., Hultman, E., Gederblad, G., Graham, T. E., 'Caffeine ingestion and muscle metabolism during prolonged exercise in humans', *American Journal of Physiology*, vol. 262, 1992.

Stremmel, W., Diede, H. E., 'Fatty acid uptake by human hepatoma cell lines represents carrier-mediated uptake process', *Biochem Biophys Acta*, vol. 1013, 1989, pp. 218–222.

Stubbs, R. J., Harbron, C. G., Murgatroyd, P. R., Prentice, A. M., 'Covert manipulation of dietary fat and energy density: effect on substrate flux and food intake in men feeding ad libitum', *American Journal of Clinical Nutrition*, vol. 62, 1995, pp. 316–329.

References

Weir, J., Noakes, T. D., Myburgh, K., Adams, B., 'A high-carbohydrate diet negates the metabolic effects of caffeine during exercise', *Medicine and Science in Sports Exercise*, vol. 19, 1987, pp. 100–105.

Yan, Z., Salmons, S., Jarvis, J., Booth, F. W., 'Increased muscle carnitine palmitoyltransferase II mRNA after increased contractile activity', *American Journal of Physiology*, vol. 68, 1995, pp. E277–E281.

INDEX

A

abdominal fat 96
adipose tissue 3, 4
adrenaline 56, 92
aerobics 102
alcohol 122–4
amino acids 32–3, 37–9, 53, 59

B

bad breath 35, 60
'bad' cholesterol 7–8, 10–11,
    12, 30
bad days 67, 71, 85
'bad' fats 5, 10
bad weeks 135–6, 140
bile 7–8
Bilsborough Fat Cost Charts
    127, 162–5

brain 26, 27–8, 39, 54–5, 59
branch chain amino acids
    37–9
breakfast 51
    alternative food choices
        117
    bad day 65–6, 69, 73
    diet eating plan 155–9
    good day 75–6, 77
    normal diet 79, 80, 81
butter 9, 10, 12

C

carbohydrates
    conversion to fat 3, 41–7,
        48
    daily requirements 26–7,
        30, 39

functions 24
and glucose production 24–6, 46
shortage of 25–6
storage 26, 27, 29
see also sugar
carnitine 57, 93
cellulite 16–17, 19, 36, 59–60, 95
cereals 149
cholesterol 4, 7–9, 10–11, 12, 30
colon cancer 29–30, 34
combining plant proteins 32
complex carbohydrates 24, 26, 39
constipation 25, 28–9
cycling as exercise 87, 88
cycling exercises 137–8

D
dairy products 20–1, 148–9
de novo lipogenesis 42–7
diabetes 47–8
dinner
alternative food choices 118
bad day 68, 69
diet eating plan 155–9
good day 77
normal diet 79, 80, 81
drinks 151

E
eating before training 97–9, 106
eating out 120–1
eating patterns
bad day 65–9, 73–4

good day 75–8
normal day 79–83
eating plans 115–16, 154–9
eicosanoids 11, 12
empty calories 122–3
energy cost of food 64–85, 148–53
energy cost of storage 27, 29, 35–7, 55–6, 59
enzymes 4
epinephrine 56, 92, 96
essential fatty acids (EFAs) 5–7, 11, 13
exercise
adaptation to 96–7
best time for 54–5, 57, 97–9, 106
and cellulite reduction 95
cycling exercises 137–8
duration of 89, 94, 104, 106, 128–35
eating before 97–9, 106
and fat banks 71, 74, 78, 80, 82
for fat loss 69, 71–2, 87–9, 127
and fat-stripping diet 74–5, 126–39
in the heat 105
and high-fat diet 84
intensity of 87–94
metabolism of 93, 105–6
principles of 89
spot reduction 96
without diet 136–7, 138
see also specific activities
exercise equipment 15, 94–5
exercise pyramid 138

F
fad diets 83–4
fast foods 152–3
fat
  from carbohydrate
    conversion 3, 41–7, 48
  cellulite 16–17, 19, 36,
    59–60, 95
  daily needs 2, 13, 26, 70
  as energy source 53, 54–5,
    70
  energy yield per gram 2
  potential cost of 69
  release from fat cell 50,
    55–7, 58, 63, 90–1, 93, 97
  risks of high intake 14–15
  types in body 3–5
  types in food 5–14
fat banks
  bad day 71, 74, 78
  and exercise 71, 74, ,78, 80,
    82
  good day 78
  normal day 80, 82
fat burning 35, 123
  and fitness levels 96–7
  and insulin 50–1, 54, 57–8,
    61, 63, 98, 99
  specific exercises 100–4
fat-burning foods 18–19
fat cost charts 162–5
fat loss 128–9
  assessing 143–4, 160–4
  myths about 94–5
fat-soluble vitamins 3, 4
fat storage 46–7, 53, 63
  and consumption 69–70,
    83

  energy used in 27, 55–6
  sites 3, 4, 15–17, 55
fat-stripping 50–1
  best time for 54–5, 57, 63
  exercises for 86–106
fat-stripping diet 108–9,
    145–6
  alcohol 122–4
  alternative food choices
    116–20
  bad weeks 135–6, 140
  eating out 120–1
  eating plans 115–16,
    154–9
  and exercise 111, 126–38,
    141
  format 115
  maximum fat intake 110,
    112, 126
  motivation 140–6
  night off 121–2
  planning 142–3
  principles of 110–15
  weekends 122
fat surplus point 82
fatty acids 5, 7, 11, 13, 35,
    56–7
fibre 28, 29–31, 34
fish 12, 149–50
fitness and fat burning 96–7
food combining 37
free-fatty acids 56–7
fructose 47
fruit 151

G
glucagon 55, 56–7
gluconeogenesis 35–6

glucose
  from carbohydrates 24–6, 46
  as energy source 25, 27–8, 39, 52, 54
  and glucagon 55, 56–7
  and insulin 30, 50–1, 52, 53–4
  from proteins 35–7
  storage 25, 42, 52
glucose sparing 55
glycogen 25
golf 103
'good' cholesterol 7–8, 10
'good' fats 5, 10, 13, 83
'good' oils 12
grains 149
grazing 115, 119, 120

H
HDL (high-density lipoprotein) 7–8, 10
heart disease 8, 10, 12, 14, 34
hidden fats 10, 67, 68, 72
high-carbohydrate diet 52, 53–4, 60, 61
high-fat diet 60, 83–4
high-fibre diet 31, 34
high-intensity exercise 88–9, 93–4, 95, 102, 103, 106
high-protein diet 34–7, 61
hormones 4–5, 6, 7, 15–16

I
inert proteins 31
insulin
  and blood glucose 50–3
  and diabetes 30, 47, 54
  and fat burning 50–1, 54, 57–8, 61, 63, 98, 99
  and high-carbohydrate diet 52, 53–4, 61
  and high-protein diet 35, 61–3
isoleucine 38

J
jogging 58, 66, 87–8, 89, 100

K
ketone bodies 35

L
LDL (low-density lipoproteins) 7–8, 10–11, 12, 30
leucine 38
'light' foods 19–22
linoleic acid 6
linolenic acid 6
lipid see fat
lipolysis 50, 55–7, 58, 63, 90–1, 93, 97
lipoproteins 4–5, 7–8
liver 4–5, 7, 52
long-chain fatty acids 12
low-fat foods 15, 19–22, 74
low-intensity exercise 57, 87, 88–9, 90–1, 95, 106, 137
lunch 51–2
  alternative food choices 117–18
  bad day 66–7, 69
  diet eating plan 155–9
  good day 76, 77
  normal diet 79, 80, 81

M

macronutrients 52

malonly-Co-A (enzyme) 93

margarine 9, 10–11, 12

meat 149–50

medium-intensity exercise 88, 91–2, 94, 137

men

bad food day 65–9

daily carbohydrate needs 26–7

daily fat consumption 84, 136

daily fat needs 2, 13, 70, 129

daily kJ consumption 43

daily protein needs 33

diet eating plan 154–9

exercise plans 133–5

fat loss 129

fat storage sites 15–16

fat surplus point 82

fat use chart 160–2

normal food day 81–2

metabolic fats 3, 4

metabolism 4, 51, 73

of exercise 93, 105–6

mitochondria 57, 93, 97

mono-unsaturated fat 9, 12–13

motivation 140–6

muscle mass increase 38, 104, 105

muscle mass loss 36, 59–60

N

nervous system 26, 27–8, 54–5

not eating and weight loss 58–60

O

oils 2, 12, 13–14

olive oil 5, 6, 9, 12–13, 14

omega-3 fatty acids 11, 12

omega-3 fish oils 12

osteoporosis 58

overeating 43–4

overweight, Australian statistics 14–15

oxidation 35, 57–60, 63, 90–1, 96–7, 123

P

personal trainer 141

phytic acid 31

polyunsaturated fat 9, 10–11, 13

power walking 89

protein

biological value of 32–3, 36–7

daily requirement 26, 33, 34, 39

energy cost of storage 35–7, 59

as energy source 35–7, 59

functions 31–2

high-protein diet 34–7, 39, 61

and insulin 35, 61–3

produced in body 34

sources 31

supplements 37–9

protein quality 32–3

protein turnover 34

puffing 87–8, 89, 90, 96, 102
pump classes 103
pyramid cycle 138

R
resistance training 26, 104

S
satiety 26, 29, 34, 39
saturated fat 9, 10
simple carbohydrates 24, 26
snacks
    alternative food choices
       115, 119, 120
    bad day 66, 69, 73
    diet eating plan 155–9
    energy costs of 151
    good day 76, 77
spinning 103
sports amenorrhoea 58
spot reduction 96
steroids 5
storage fats 3, 83
stroke 8, 14
structural fats 3
sucrose 47
sugar
    conversion to fat 41–7, 48
    and diabetes 47–8
surplus fat 2
swimming 100–2

T
tennis 103
thermic effect of food 27
training *see* exercise

trans-fatty acids 11–12
transit time of food 30
transport fats 3, 4–5

V
valine 38
vegetables 11, 151
vitamins 4, 31

W
walking 57, 66, 87, 88–9, 92,
    100, 127, 128–9, 137,
    145–6
weight loss
    and high-fibre foods 29, 39
    by not eating 58–60
    plateau phase 144
weight training 26, 104
women
    bad food day 73–4
    cellulite 16–17, 95
    daily carbohydrate need
       26–7
    daily fat consumption
       51–3, 84, 136
    daily fat need 2, 13, 70, 128
    daily protein need 33
    diet eating plan 154–9
    exercise plans 130–2
    fat loss 128–9
    fat storage sites 15, 16–17
    fat surplus point 82
    fat use chart 160–2
    high-protein diet 36
    normal food day 79–81
    sports amenorrhoea 58